Advance Praise for
Integrated Care: Working at the Interface of Primary Care and Behavioral Health

"In the rapidly changing world of health care, this book provides a road map in a critical area of need, the role of the psychiatrists and other prescribers in these integrated systems of care. Dr. Raney and her colleagues represent the leaders in this transforming part of medicine, and this book is must reading for anyone leading these emerging systems of care. It covers the full continuum of integration and is an essential guide for practice and also potential research directions."

> Joan Kenerson King, APRN, BC, Senior Integration Consultant, The National Council for Behavioral Health

"*Integrated Care* is a well-edited, authoritative resource for clinicians working at the interface of primary care and behavioral health. Lori Raney, an acknowledged expert in integrated care, has edited chapters from an outstanding array of the leading voices in the field, who present the evidence for integrated care and provide guidance for psychiatric practice in general medical settings. The book is an essential tool for psychiatrists who wish to expand their practice opportunities in the future."

> Howard H. Goldman, M.D., Ph.D., Professor of Psychiatry, University of Maryland School of Medicine, Baltimore, Maryland

"*Integrated Care* is a much needed comprehensive review of essential psychiatric practice in the context of 21st century health reform. By providing models of collaborative mental health care in primary care settings and primary care in mental health settings, this volume addresses the clinical realities and public health imperatives of recognizing and treating comorbid psychiatric and general medical illness. Psychiatric trainees, early-career psychiatrists, and everyone in the mental health field will find this of immense value."

> Steven S. Sharfstein, M.D., President and CEO, Sheppard Pratt, Baltimore, Maryland

"Health reform represents great potential for changes in the delivery of health care. Integrated care as one component is a develo̶p̶i̶n̶g̶ ̶'̶ e embracing increasing segments of mer̶ ̶ ̶ ̶ ̶ ̶ ̶ ̶ ̶ ̶ ̶ ̶ ̶ ̶ ̶ here is considerable evidence pointing t̶c̶ ̶ ̶ ̶ ̶ ̶ ̶ ̶ ated care. Its value is being increasingly̶ ̶ ̶ ̶ ̶ ̶ ̶ ̶ ̶ ̶ sys-tems around the country. Dr. Raney̶ ̶ ̶ ̶ ̶ ̶ ̶ ̶ ̶ ̶ ̶ the array of issues, ranging from mecha̶i̶ ̶ ̶ ̶ ̶ ̶ ̶ ̶ de-velopment of an adequate workforce̶,̶ ̶ ̶ ̶ ̶ ̶ ̶ ̶ ̶ ̶ s̶ ̶ ̶ ̶ ̶ ̶ ̶ ̶ liability. For all interested in the broad sweep of mental health care and its evolution in conjunction with health reform, this superb text brings comprehensive information and helps signal a dramatic movement in the history of mental health care."

Herbert Pardes, M.D., Executive Vice Chairman of the Board of Trustees, New York-Presbyterian

"What comes to mind is the Rosetta Stone. That single ancient rock is remembered today because of its value in translating and sorting out a variety of languages. With *Integrated Care: Working at the Interface of Primary Care and Behavioral Health*, Lori Raney has skillfully brought together the multiple languages and vast experience with integrated care and put it into one very useful document that is both scholarly and extremely practical. I have personally been involved with the design and execution of over three different integrated care projects here at Johns Hopkins. This book is going to become a mandatory read for all our project staff. It is a great asset to the field. Thank you, Lori and all, for assembling such a valuable group of authors to provide such a valuable book."

Anita Everett, M.D., DFAFA, Division Director Community and General Psychiatry, Johns Hopkins Bayview Medical Center, Baltimore, Maryland

"Dr. Raney has assembled the best available talent from a wide array of disciplines to build the definitive text of integrated behavioral health, with particular relevance to the roles and contributions of psychiatrists. From the first page to the last, it is clear that her level of expertise and experience informs a practical yet thoroughly scientific treatment of this ever-evolving model of practice. …Case examples bring to life the unique skills and capabilities necessary for optimal implementation of integrated behavioral health care in the primary care setting. This text is a remarkable achievement that will become the standard referral resource for clinicians in new and established integrated behavioral health programs."

James R. Rundell, M.D., Department of Psychiatry, Veterans Administration Medical Center, Minneapolis, Minnesota

"Integrated care is no longer a research subject, waiting for data to support its use. In this book, written by an all-star group of authors, Dr. Raney has assembled a guide to operationalizing a new way for psychiatrists to function in both primary and behavioral health care settings. The Affordable Care Act has the potential to provide care to many people who now have no such access. That goal will require that we learn how to integrate care and collaborate with our colleagues in a variety of settings. This book is required reading for those who will participate in 21st century psychiatry."

Philip R. Muskin, M.D., Professor of Psychiatry at CUMC and Chief of Service: Consultation-Liaison Psychiatry, New York-Presbyterian Hospital/Columbia University Medical Center

"As a psychiatrist who has spent most of his career training public psychiatrists, I found the chapter 'Training Psychiatrists for Integrated Care' particularly informative. The authors emphasize that psychiatrists working in integrated career need to focus on indirect care with much of the communication occurring via telephone, televideo, or electronic forms such as e-mail, text, and electronic medical records. The approach utilizes population-based care and measurement-based treatment with regular use of screening instruments: depending on electronic databases to track key clinical and quality-of-care outcomes of a specific population of patients to determine which patients need 'step-up' care; 'ruling out' high-risk conditions and trusting the team to initiate a preliminary treatment plan even in the absence of a 'perfect' diagnosis; delivering brief behavioral interventions that have been proven effective in primary care settings."

Jules M. Ranz, M.D., Clinical Professor of Psychiatry and Director, Public Psychiatry Fellowship, New York State Psychiatric Institute/Columbia, University Medical Center

"Dr. Lori Raney's *Integrated Care: Working at the Interface of Primary Care and Behavioral Health* is an invaluable and catalytic tool for psychiatric physicians, primary care colleagues, and the collaborative primary care/behavioral health team to seize the opportunities stimulated by the Affordable Care Act and the evolving new models of populations' health and team-based care. It is well grounded in Dr. Raney's, hands-on clinical experience with primary care/behavioral health collaboration in the state of Colorado, and it offers a clear, concise, and pragmatic path for its adoption and implementation in other settings. I highly recommend it to all interested in better navigating and engaging in the evolving American health system."

Eliot Sorel, M.D., Clinical Professor of Global Health & Psychiatry, The George Washington University, Washington, D.C.; APA Board of Trustees Work Group on Health Reform, APA Council on Health Systems & Financing

"This book is much needed. It introduces a crucial member of the team, the consulting psychiatrist, to the collaborative care process in integrated primary care. It does a first-rate job of introducing psychiatrists to both the routines of practice and to the spirit of multidisciplinary team work on which the success of primary care behavioral health integration depends."

Alexander Blount, Ed.D., Director, Center for Integrated Primary Care, and Professor of Family Medicine and Psychiatry, University of Massachusetts Medical School, and Director of Behavioral Science, Department of Family Medicine and Community Health

"Lori Raney's edited volume is the answer to the question we are all asking—how do we effectively integrate psychiatric practice with primary care? The experts in this book describe a critical new role for psychiatrists, show us the data, describe the core principles, and detail the new attitudes, skills, and behaviors needed to collaborate effectively with primary care providers. This will be an essential resource for the next generation of residents and other psychiatrists ready to step into the future."

Richard F. Summers, M.D., Clinical Professor of Psychiatry and Co-Director of Residency Training, Perelman School of Medicine of the University of Pennsylvania; Past-President, American Association of Directors of Psychiatry Residency Training; Chair, Council on Medical Education and Lifelong Learning, American Psychiatric Association

"*Integrated Care: Working at the Interface of Primary Care and Behavioral Health* is an excellent and timely book. Its depiction of team-based care, roles for behavioral health professionals, primary care physicians, and psychiatrists, and changes necessary for training and practice is comprehensive and impressive. The book contains an outstanding chapter on integration in pediatrics and child mental health. If you believe that integrated care is best for our patients and our practice as I do, this book will help you transform your care of your patients."

John Sargent, M.D., Director, Division of Child and Adolescent Psychiatry, Tufts Medical School, Professor of Psychiatry and Pediatrics, Tufts University School of Medicine, Boston, Massachusetts

"Teamwork is essential for us to treat patients as whole people, with heart and mind, body and soul, all connected. This book provides a strong evidence base for the bidirectional integration of primary care and behavioral health in a collaborative care model, with practical strategies for implementing these models and for training a new generation of professionals to practice psychiatry as a team sport in the 21st century."

George Rust, M.D., M.P.H., FAAFP, FACPM, Professor of Family Medicine and Co-Director, National Center for Primary Care, Morehouse School of Medicine, Atlanta, Georgia

"Dr. Raney and her colleagues have been able to distill technique and evidential knowledge into a highly practical, eminently readable, as well as clearly groundbreaking, book that assists clinicians and administrators as they move into psychiatry's future. It will be read, read again, and then again, as an essential guide to plan, implement, and practice in collaborative care settings. Primary care providers will also find *Integrated Care* very helpful as they themselves orient their own work in new collaborative contexts."

Hunter L. McQuistion, M.D., Clinical Associate Professor of Psychiatry, New York University School of Medicine; Immediate Past President, American Association of Community Psychiatrists

"*Integrated Care: Working at the Interface of Primary Care and Behavioral Health* is sure to be a bedrock resource in what is one of the most rapidly growing and integral aspects of health care today. It is clear that our current 'dis-integrated' health care system is broken, driving us bankrupt, and leaving millions to suffer with untreated mental illness. There is no viable path forward without integration. Regardless of where you live in the health care ecosystem, Dr. Raney leverages her proven track record of 'on-the-ground' system transformation and calls on her friends—who also happen to be the best of the best—to assemble a map that points the way forward and shows us all how to catch up. This book is a must-have for leaders, administrators, and clinicians alike."

John Santopietro, M.D., FAPA, Chief Clinical Officer of Behavioral Health, Carolinas HealthCare System, Charlotte, North Carolina

"With the advent of health care reform, collaborative care is fast becoming an extremely important mental health service delivery model. Psychiatrists must have a seat at the table in developing and implementing integrated care models across a variety of health care settings. *Integrated Care: Working at the Interface of Primary Care and Behavioral Health* is prerequisite reading for any psychiatrist hoping to make a significant contribution to the discussion and practice of integrated care."

Ruth Shim, M.D., M.P.H., Associate Professor, Department of Psychiatry and Behavioral Sciences Associate, and Director of Behavioral Health, National Center for Primary Care Morehouse School of Medicine, Atlanta, Georgia

INTEGRATED CARE

Working at the Interface of Primary Care and Behavioral Health

INTEGRATED CARE

Working at the Interface of Primary Care and Behavioral Health

Edited by

Lori E. Raney, M.D.

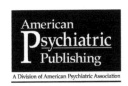

American **Psychiatric** Publishing

A Division of American Psychiatric Association

Washington, DC
London, England

If you would like to buy between 25 and 99 copies of this or any other American Psychiatric Publishing title, you are eligible for a 20% discount; please contact Customer Service at appi@psych.org or 800-368-5777. If you wish to buy 100 or more copies of the same title, please e-mail us at bulksales@psych.org for a price quote.

Manufactured in the United States of America on acid-free paper
18   17   16   15   5   4   3   2
First Edition

Typeset in Trade Gothic LT Std and Warnock Pro.

American Psychiatric Publishing
A Division of American Psychiatric Association
1000 Wilson Boulevard
Arlington, VA 22209-3901
www.appi.org

Library of Congress Cataloging-in-Publication Data
Integrated care (Raney)
   Integrated care : working at the interface of primary care and behavioral health / edited by Lori E. Raney.—First edition.
      p. ; cm.
   Includes bibliographical references and index.
   ISBN 978-1-58562-480-5 (pbk. : alk. paper)
   I. Raney, Lori E., 1960– editor. II. American Psychiatric Association, issuing body. III. Title.
   [DNLM: 1. Delivery of Health Care, Integrated. 2. Mental Health Services—organization & administration. 3. Continuity of Patient Care—organization & administration. 4. Primary Health Care—organization & administration. WM 30.1]
   RC455
   362.19689—dc23
                              2014019005

British Library Cataloguing in Publication Data
A CIP record is available from the British Library.

CONTENTS

Section I
Behavioral Health in Primary Care Settings

Section II
Primary Care in Behavioral Health Settings

Contributors

D. Anton Bland, M.D.
Consultation-Liaison Psychiatrist, Alameda Health Systems, Oakland, California

Lydia Chwastiak, M.D., M.P.H.
Associate Professor, Department of Psychiatry and Behavioral Health Sciences, University of Washington, Harborview Medical Center, Seattle, Washington

Benjamin G. Druss, M.D., M.P.H.
Rosalynn Carter Chair in Mental Health, Department of Health Policy and Management, Rollins School of Public Health, Emory University, Atlanta, Georgia

Robert Hilt, M.D.
Medical Director, Partnership Access Line, Seattle Children's Hospital; Associate Professor, Department of Psychiatry, University of Washington, Seattle, Washington

Wayne Katon, M.D.
Professor of Psychiatry and Behavioral Sciences, Director, Division of Health Services and Psychiatric Epidemiology, and Adjunct Professor, Department of Health Services, University of Washington School of Medicine, Seattle, Washington

John S. Kern, M.D.
Chief Medical Officer, Regional Mental Health Center, Merrillville, Indiana

Kristen Lambert, J.D., M.S.W., LICSW, FASHRM
Vice President Risk Management, AWAC Services Company, Boston, Massachusetts

Gina Lasky, Ph.D.
Project Manager, Health Management Associates, Denver, Colorado

Joseph Parks, M.D.
Distinguished Professor of Science, Missouri Institute of Mental Health, University of Missouri, St. Louis, Missouri

Marcella Pascualy, M.D.
Associate Professor of Psychiatry and Behavioral Sciences, VA Puget Sound Health Care System, Seattle, Washington

Lori Raney, M.D.
Medical Director, Axis Health System, Durango, Colorado; Owner, Collaborative Care Consulting, Dolores, Colorado

Anna H. Ratzliff, M.D., Ph.D.
Assistant Professor, Department of Psychiatry and Behavioral Sciences, University of Washington, Seattle, Washington

Barry Sarvet, M.D.
Chief of Child and Adolescent Psychiatry and Vice Chair, Baystate Health, Springfield, Massachusetts; Associate Clinical Professor, Department of Psychiatry, Tufts School of Medicine, Boston, Massachusetts

Clare Scott, LCSW
Associate, Collaborative Care Consulting, Lafayette, Colorado

Jürgen Unützer, M.D., M.P.H., M.A.
Professor and Chair, Department of Psychiatry and Behavioral Sciences, Adjunct Professor, Health Services and Global Health, Director, Division of Integrated Care and Public Health, and Director, AIMS (Advancing Integrated Mental Health Solutions) Center, University of Washington, Seattle, Washington

Erik R. Vanderlip, M.D., M.P.H.
Assistant Professor, Department of Psychiatry, University of Oklahoma School of Community Medicine, Tulsa, Oklahoma

Martha C. Ward, M.D.
Assistant Professor, Department of Psychiatry and Behavioral Sciences, Department of Medicine, Emory University, Atlanta, Georgia

Disclosure of Competing Interests

None of the contributors to this book have indicated competing interests to disclose during the year preceding manuscript submission.

Foreword

Wayne Katon, M.D.

Over the last two decades, epidemiologic studies have shown that mental health disorders (largely depressive, anxiety, and substance abuse disorders) occur in approximately 20%–25% of primary care patients and that quality of mental health care is poor and mental health outcomes are problematic (Seelig and Katon 2008). This results in unnecessary suffering of patients and their families, as well as high costs to both employers and the health care system. Epidemiologic studies have also shown that patients with major depression (who are largely treated in primary care) as well as those with severe mental illness (who largely receive care in community mental health centers) have high rates of medical comorbidity and often have major deficits in being able to access primary care and specialty medical care, as well as problems affording disease-control medications for chronic medical illnesses (Bradford et al. 2008). Recent studies have shown that patients with depression as well as those with serious mental illness (SMI) are dying about 10–20 years earlier from chronic medical illnesses (Druss et al. 2011).

Fortunately, researchers have developed health service models of care that have been shown to improve quality and outcomes of mental and physical health care in primary care systems, as well as medical care for patients with SMI in community mental health systems. In primary care systems, a recent meta-analysis of 79 studies found that collaborative depression and anxiety care models significantly improved quality of care and depressive and anxiety outcomes compared to usual primary care (Archer et al. 2012). Several recent primary care–based studies have also shown that multicondition collaborative care approaches can improve both depression and medical disease control for patients with major depression and poorly controlled medical illnesses, such as cardiovascular disease and diabetes (Bogner et al. 2012; Katon et al. 2010). Recent studies have tested models that integrated primary care services into care of patients with SMI treated in community mental health centers and have found improved quality of medical care and clinical outcomes compared to usual care (Druss et al. 2010).

This state-of-the-art book describes in careful detail the key components of these integrated models of care, evidence of their effectiveness, and the change in roles for a psychiatrist who becomes involved in these models of care. Key concepts such as population-based care, measurement-based care, and stepped care are explained and highlighted. The book also emphasizes how health reform initiatives are stimulating rapid dissemination of these models of care. The authors of these chapters, such as Jürgen Unützer, Lori Raney, John Kern, Ben Druss, Lydia Chwastiak, and Joe Parks, are leaders in this field and are directing dissemination efforts in large systems of care throughout the United States. Psychiatrists have an important potential role to play in aiding these dissemination efforts, and this book should help psychiatrists understand the key changes in usual care that will be important to make to develop effective integrated models of care.

The book also covers the issue of workforce training. We need to develop a cadre of psychiatrists, as well as care managers and researchers, who are trained in integrated care models and who can be instrumental in staffing the clinics that are integrating these models, as well as study the cost-effectiveness of these changes in care. Therefore, training programs will need to be integrated into psychiatric residencies as well as social work and nurse training so that future health care systems have professional staff who are equipped to fill these roles. We also need fellowship training in this interface of psychiatry and medicine so that researchers can continue to increase the knowledge base regarding the maladaptive effects of comorbid psychiatric and medical illness, as well as continue to develop and shape the most effective models of care.

In summary, this book provides state-of-the art data on the importance of developing integrated models of care, describes in detail the key components of these models, and describes the ongoing dissemination efforts in multiple states. It should be required reading for psychiatric residents and other professionals who want to help develop and disseminate these models of care in their own health care systems.

REFERENCES

Archer J, Bower P, Gilbody S, et al: Collaborative care for depression and anxiety problems. Cochrane Database of Systematic Reviews 2012, Issue 10. Art. No.: CD006525. DOI: 10.1002/14651858.CD006525.pub2.

Bogner HR, Morales KH, de Vries HF, et al: Integrated management of type 2 diabetes mellitus and depression treatment to improve medication adherence: a randomized controlled trial. Ann Fam Med 10:15–22, 2012

Bradford DW, Kim MM, Braxton LE, et al: Access to medical care among persons with psychotic and major affective disorders. Psychiatr Serv 59:847–852, 2008

Druss BG, von Esenwein SA, Compton MT, et al: A randomized trial of medical care management for community mental health settings: the Primary Care Access, Referral, and Evaluation (PCARE) study. Am J Psychiatry 167:151–159, 2010

Druss BG, Zhao L, Von Esenwein S, et al: Understanding excess mortality in persons with mental illness: 17-year follow up of a nationally representative US survey. Med Care 49:599–604, 2011

Katon WJ, Lin EH, Von Korff M, et al: Collaborative care for patients with depression and chronic illnesses. N Engl J Med 363:2611–2620, 2010

Seelig MD, Katon W: Gaps in depression care: why primary care physicians should hone their depression screening, diagnosis, and management skills. J Occup Environ Med 50:451–458, 2008

Preface

Lori Raney, M.D.

The integration of primary care and behavioral health presents new opportunities for psychiatrists to have a major impact at all levels of the triple aim in health care: improving outcomes, containing costs, and enhancing the patient experience of care. Evidence-based models of collaborative care (CC) were tested over a decade ago while looking for better treatment of depression in elderly patients in primary care settings but failed to be implemented, mostly because of funding barriers. Newer models are emerging with the news of the 25-year reduced life expectancy for those with serious mental illness (SMI), and they offer the promise of addressing the health disparity in this group. The passage of the Patient Protection and Affordable Care Act in 2010, with the full implementation of all major components in 2014, provides health care insurance for a greater portion of the population, requirements for more effective and coordinated care, and incentives to contain costs.

This book aims to provide psychiatrists with additional skills to complement their traditional way of training and practice in order to work in this new health care arena. To be successful, it is important to understand that a fundamental shift is under way for all of health care that places an emphasis on the health of populations rather than the individual patient. It is a shift in thinking about denominators (a defined population of patients) instead of numerators (just those patients who present for treatment). The new models of integrated care presented in this book have this concept of population-based care at their core and present a change in how psychiatry and all of medicine will be expected to approach health care delivery moving forward. It is this important revision that allows psychiatric expertise to be distributed across a broader population, which is central to improving outcomes.

The information presented in these chapters allows the practicing psychiatrist and those still in training to develop an essential skill set, whether they are designing, working within, teaching, or trying to sell an integrated care program to a health care system. These chapters cover the evidence base, business case, inner workings of the models, methods of teaching integrated care, improving the health status of patients with SMI, liability, and more, while carefully describing the specific tasks and skills the psychiatrists need to feel competent and confident in this new field of expertise. Each chapter repeats the theme of a set of core principles of effective collaborative care, which serve as a guide for the structure and provision of care for the varying models regardless of the setting. Throughout the text are numerous examples of the impact psychiatrists can have in all areas of the triple aim. Staff and patient experiences are an integral part of the chapters, as are detailed case vignettes further describing the concepts. The book is divided into two sections: Section I covers improving the detection and treatment of behavioral health conditions by integrating behavioral health services into primary care settings, and Section II addresses improving the health status of the population with SMI by integrating primary care into behavioral health treatment.

LEXICON

The terms *integrated care* and *collaborative care* are often used interchangeably and essentially imply a similar delivery system. One way to think about this is that systems integrate (administrative structures, billing and finance, electronic medical records, etc.) and people collaborate (provide the actual health care in teams of professionals working together). The Agency for Healthcare Research and Quality has developed a lexicon and definition of integrated care (http://integrationacademy.ahrq.gov/lexicon) that provide a helpful starting point.

> The care that results from a practice team of primary care and behavioral health clinicians, working together with patients and families, using a systematic and cost-effective approach to provide patient-centered care for a defined population. This care may address mental health and substance abuse conditions, health behaviors (including their contribution to chronic medical illnesses), life stressors and crises, stress-related physical symptoms, and ineffective patterns of health care utilization.

In this book, the terms *integrated care* and *collaborative care* are used interchangeably, and the term *behavioral health* is used to imply both mental health and substance use services. Another area where terminology is used interchangeably is when indicating the role in the primary care setting of the nonmedical behavioral health provider. In the original studies, these professionals were called "care managers," but as the model was replicated, some organizations started to use *behavioral health provider* or *behavioral health consultant. Behavioral health provider* and *care manager* are the terms used in this text. Last, it is well understood that a variety of "psychiatric prescribers" are working in these settings, and the terms *consultant psychiatrist* and *consultant psychiatric provider* are both used throughout.

The Center for Integrated Health Solutions developed the Standard Framework for Levels of Integrated Healthcare (www.integration.samhsa.gov/resource/standard-framework-for-levels-of-integrated-healthcare). This is designed to help organizations to develop a common language for integration and to understand where they are along the continuum of collaboration and where they may want to be in the future. The framework is divided into three categories called coordinated, colocated, and integrated, with each subdivided into two additional sections for a total of six levels of integration. This framework can be used to help organizations in assessing and planning their integration efforts, and it describes the advantages of each category.

SECTION I

Section I covers the integration of behavioral health into primary care settings to improve access to behavioral health services and reach a population of patients who require more effective care. Chapter 1 ("Evidence Base and Core Principles") details the evidence base and cost-effectiveness of current models of CC and introduces the five core principles of CC. Chapter 2 ("The Collaborative Care Team in Action") provides a detailed description of the core features of the CC model and introduces TEMP-A as an acronym for remembering the core principles. Staff and patient experiences along with case vignettes are interwoven throughout this chapter and others in the book. Chapter 3 ("Role of the Consulting Psychiatrist") describes the specific tasks of the consulting psychiatrist, with a focus on leadership approaches to help teams utilize the unique training psychiatrists bring to straddle the cultures of primary care and behavioral health more successfully. Chapter 4 ("Child and Adolescent Psychiatry in Integrated Settings") takes a detailed look at providing CC services for children, an area less researched but ripe with emerging models and interest and a more significant shortage of psychiatric professionals. Detailed case vignettes offer a window into this area, which is important for psychiatrists trained in adult psychiatry because they are often asked as part of their consultation duties to provide input on children and adolescents being treated in primary care. Chapter 5 ("Risk Management and Liability Issues in Integrated Care") covers major liability concerns when providing indirect consultation and caseload-based review. These are necessary to fulfill the intent of the CC model but present some uncharted territory in the malpractice world. Chapter 6 ("Training Psychiatrists for Integrated Care") wraps up this section with a detailed description of how to proceed with training the workforce to practice in CC settings, with an emphasis on how to meet the Accreditation Council for Graduate Medical Education–American Board of Psychiatry and Neurology psychiatry milestones requirements.

SECTION II

Section II describes the current landscape in the public behavioral health sector and ways to improve the health status of the population with SMI by describing emerging models of integrating primary care principles into behavioral health settings. While this area does not have the robust evidence base seen for the CC models presented in Section I, several models are showing promise, and practices across the country have implemented various ways to address this physical health disparity. Chapter 7 ("The Case for Primary Care in Public Mental Health Settings") outlines the problem of the health burden experienced by the population with SMI, exploring the social determinants of health and outlining new responsibilities for psychiatrists to assume greater oversight of patients' total health care. Chapter 8 ("Providing Primary Care in Behavioral Health Settings") is written by a Primary Behavioral Health Care Integration project grantee and gives a detailed description of the core features of this model, which brings primary care services into behavioral health settings. Chapter 9 ("Behavioral Health Homes") describes the requirements of Section 2703 (of the Patient Protection and Affordable Care Act) Medicaid State Plan Amendments for behavioral health homes using the most advanced program in Missouri as a case study. Chapter 10 ("Management of Leading Risk Factors for Cardiovascular Disease") follows the treatment of a patient with schizophrenia called "B.H." through the course of addressing his chronic medical conditions that contribute to his increased risk of dying 25 years prematurely. The treatment of each of these preventable risk factors (dyslipidemia, hypertension, obesity, diabetes, smoking) is discussed with evidence-based care guidelines that could be followed by a practicing psychiatrist in partnership with a primary care provider.

CONCLUSION

This book is intended to provide trainees and practicing psychiatrists and others with practical approaches to collaborative care in a variety of settings. The information presented in these chapters will provide ample guidance for the psychiatric provider to work competently in the new health care arena.

Acknowledgments

I would like to thank Jürgen Unützer, M.D., Ben Druss, M.D., Wayne Katon, M.D., Roger Kathol M.D., and Joe Parks, M.D., for sharing their experiences and expertise with me over the years and for their generous participation in this project. My colleagues John Kern, M.D., and Anna Ratzliff, M.D., have been constant companions in the goal to train psychiatrists to do this work, and I thank them for sharing their stories with me and the readers of this book. I would also like to thank Karen Sanders at the American Psychiatric Association for her foresight in realizing that integrated care was important to our professional organization and for prompting me to become involved from within the organization.

My partners Gina Lasky, Ph.D., and Clare Scott, LCSW, have been invaluable in sharing their thoughtful understanding of the cultural differences that emerge in collaborative care settings and how to work successfully across these boundaries. Additional thanks go to Bern Heath, Ph.D., and Pam Wise-Romero, Ph.D., at Axis Health System for providing the vision and subsequent opportunity for me to explore the landscape of integrated care through hands-on experience.

I would like to thank my husband Don and daughter Elizabeth for their patience and support throughout this process. Last, I would like to extend my appreciation to the American Psychiatric Publishing staff for their guidance and support for my first-time adventure into editing.

Section I

Behavioral Health in Primary Care Settings

CHAPTER 1

 Evidence Base and Core Principles

Jürgen Unützer, M.D., M.P.H., M.A.

Anna H. Ratzliff, M.D., Ph.D.

Psychiatrists are an important component of the physician workforce in the United States, but the roughly 40,000 practicing psychiatrists are distributed unequally around the country, and the behavioral health needs of the majority of the population are more likely to be met by primary care physicians and other behavioral health professionals than by psychiatrists (Wang et al. 2005). Across the country, approximately 2 in 10 adults with common mental disorders receive care from a mental health specialist in any given year (Wang et al. 2005). Most of the treatment for these disorders is provided in primary care, where many patients do not receive sufficient doses or duration of medications. Others continue to use medications even if they are not effective for them, rather than having their treatment adjusted, because of lack of regular monitoring and clinical inertia. As a result, as few as 20% of patients started on antidepressant medications in "usual" primary care show substantial clinical improvements (Rush et al. 2004; Unützer et al. 2002).

Existing mental health care programs do not have the capacity to provide effective treatment to all patients in need, and primary care has long been recognized as the de facto location of care for most adults in the United States with common mental disorders such as depression (Regier et al. 1993; Wang et al. 2006). Primary care providers (PCPs) are well aware of the substantial challenges related to treating patients with behavioral health problems in primary care, and they report serious limitations in the support they receive from mental health specialists (Cunningham 2009). When patients are referred to mental health specialists by a PCP, almost half do not follow through with the referral (Grembowski et al. 2002), and the mean number of appointments among those who do pursue a specialty mental health referral is two visits (Simon et al. 2012).

Collaborative care (CC) is an evidence-based, systematic approach in which primary care and behavioral health providers work closely together to deliver effective treatment for depression and other common mental disorders in primary care settings. It represents one opportunity for psychiatrists to "leverage" their unique skills and reach a larger share of the millions of people living with mental health and substance abuse problems who are in need of quality care.

Effective collaboration of psychiatrists with primary care and other medical providers also creates an opportunity to provide a more patient-centered and integrated health care experience. Most patients with mental health and substance use disorders also have one or more acute or chronic medical problems, and this combination of behavioral and medical disorders can substantially worsen associated health outcomes (Moussavi et al. 2007). When behavioral health problems are not effectively treated, they can impair self-care and adherence to medical and mental health treatments, and they are associated with poor health outcomes and increased mortality. This interaction of behavioral and physical health problems at an individual and population level (Katon 2003; Moussavi et al. 2007) suggests that when psychiatrists collaborate more closely with their medical colleagues, they have a greater chance of providing care that addresses the whole spectrum of medical and behavioral health needs of patients.

In recent years, patient-centered medical homes (PCMHs) have been advocated as a way to provide better health care to populations of patients at a lower cost, and effective "medical homes" should be able to address common mental disorders such as depression (Katon and Unützer 2013). The National Committee for Quality Assurance has developed criteria for levels of adaptation of practices to the medical home concept, and these criteria require the capacity to address chronic medical conditions and common behavioral health conditions such as depression in primary care (National Committee for Quality Assurance 2011). CC offers an important opportunity for psychiatrists to become effective contributors to the care provided in these PCMHs.

EVIDENCE BASE FOR COLLABORATIVE CARE

Efforts to improve the collaboration of psychiatrists and PCPs date back to early consultation-liaison interventions and, more recently, in attempts to colocate mental health specialists within primary care clinics. Having a behavioral health provider available can improve access to mental health services in primary care, but such colocation alone has also not been found to improve patient outcomes at a population level (Uebelacker et al. 2009).

Over the past 20 years, more than 79 randomized controlled trials involving more than 24,000 participants have established a robust evidence base for an approach called "collaborative care" for common mental disorders such as depression and anxiety disorders in primary care (Archer et al. 2012; Community Preventive Services Task Force 2012; Gilbody et al. 2006a; Thota et al. 2012). Trials have been conducted in the United States, several European countries, and more recently in some low-resource and middle-income countries (Patel et al. 2013). In the United States, they have included patients in diverse health care settings, including network and staff model health systems and private and public providers, with different financing mechanisms, including fee-for-service and capitation; different practice sizes; and different patient populations, including both insured and uninsured/safety net populations. Several studies have demonstrated that CC programs are not only highly effective in safety net patients and patients from ethnic minority groups (Arean et al. 2005; Ell et al. 2009, 2010a, 2010b; Miranda et al. 2003, 2004), but they can, in fact, reduce health disparities observed in such populations. Additional studies have shown that CC can be beneficial for improving medical outcomes, such as decreasing risk for cardiovascular events (Stewart et al. 2014).

Studies have also tested CC interventions for different mental health conditions, including depression (Gilbody et al. 2006b; Simon 2009), anxiety disorders, and more serious conditions such as bipolar disorder and schizophrenia (Reilly et al. 2013; Woltmann et al. 2012). Across this extensive literature, this model has consistently demonstrated greater effectiveness than usual care (Community Preventive Services Task Force 2012; Roy-Byrne et al. 2005; Thota et al. 2012). The largest study to date, the Improving Mood—Promoting Access to Collaborative Treatment (IMPACT) trial (Unützer et al. 2002), has been recognized as an evidence-based practice by the Substance Abuse and Mental Health Services Administration's National Registry of Evidence-based Programs and Practices (http://nrepp.samhsa.gov/ViewIntervention.aspx?id=301). It has also been recommended as a "best practice" by the Surgeon General (U.S. Department of Health and Human Services, 1999), the President's New Freedom Commission on Mental Health (www.businessgrouphealth.org/toolkits/et_mentalhealth.cfm), and a number of national organizations, including the National Business Group on Health (www.businessgrouphealth.org/benefitstopics/et_mentalhealth.cfm). In a recent evidence-based practice report by the Agency for Healthcare Research and Quality that reviewed the existing literature on approaches to integration of mental health/substance abuse and primary care (www.ahrq.gov/clinic/tp/mhsapctp.htm), the IMPACT program was profiled as "the study with the strongest results" (Butler et al. 2008). Figure 1–1 summarizes the studies through 2011 that met the authors' inclusion criteria for "collaborative chronic care models" (Woltmann et al. 2012).

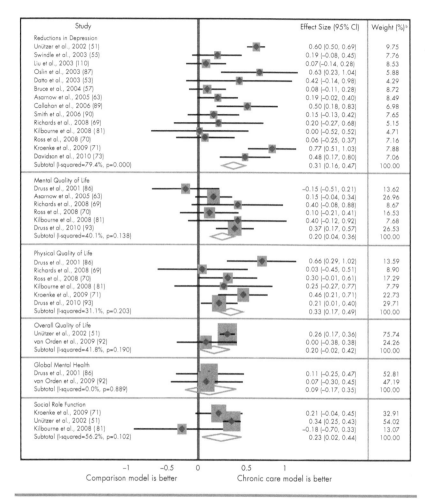

FIGURE 1–1.   Meta-analysis of clinical outcomes.

The individual comparisons extracted for these meta-analyses reflect data from the longest time interval for a given trial. The individual comparisons at these longest time points may or may not have been significantly different but were extracted for meta-analyses as the most rigorous test of the model. In complementary fashion, the systematic review results report the planned analyses as reported in each given trial, which typically included repeated-measures analyses that incorporated tests of change over time between the chronic care model and the control condition.

Weights are from random-effects analysis. CI = confidence interval.

Source.   Reprinted from Woltmann E, Grogan-Kaylor A, Perron B, et al.: "Comparative effectiveness of collaborative chronic care models for mental health conditions across primary, specialty, and behavioral health care settings: systematic review and meta-analysis." *American Journal of Psychiatry* 169(8):790–804, 2012. Used with permission. Copyright © 2012 American Psychiatric Association.

Recent studies have also shown that "multicondition collaborative care" can improve outcomes for both depression and other chronic illnesses, such as cardiovascular disease and diabetes (Bogner et al. 2012; Katon et al. 2010). Called TEAMcare, this evidence-based model is being disseminated in clinics across the nation and in other countries as well. This approach demonstrated clinically significant improvements in HbA1c measure for diabetes, systolic blood pressure, low-density lipoprotein cholesterol, and depression scores (Katon et al. 2010).

SATISFACTION WITH THE COLLABORATIVE CARE MODEL

Last, there is both patient and provider satisfaction with the CC model. Patient satisfaction is very reassuring, with 76% of depressed older adults reporting "excellent" or "very good" satisfaction with care at 3 and 12 months (Unützer et al. 2002). In addition, PCP satisfaction with the model is also encouraging, with 90% of participants reporting satisfaction with depression care management after implementation of a primary care–based CC program (Levine et al. 2005).

Example of Patient Satisfaction With Collaborative Care

I really liked having all my care in my main doctor's office. When I was so depressed and anxious, I don't think I would have made it to another site to get help. My care manager and doctor have helped me so much. Now, I am in school and looking forward to starting an internship to become a medical assistant.

Patient in CC practice, Washington

Example of PCP Satisfaction With Collaborative Care

It helps to have somebody who has time to really fully assess a person's symptoms and get the correct diagnosis and then work with a psychiatric consultant to get the best treatment plan.

PCP in CC practice, Washington

COST-EFFECTIVENESS OF COLLABORATIVE CARE

In addition to the robust findings related to effectiveness, several studies have demonstrated that CC is more cost-effective than usual care (Gilbody et al. 2006a; Glied et al. 2010). Depression and anxiety disorders can increase overall health care costs by 50%–100%, especially in patients with multiple chronic medical disorders (Katon et al. 2003; Simon et al. 1995; Unützer et al. 1997). Several evaluations have demonstrated that CC is associated with cost savings. Long-term (4-year) cost analyses from the IMPACT study found that patients in the CC intervention arm had substantially lower overall health care costs than those in usual care (Unützer et al. 2008). An initial investment in CC of $522 resulted in net cost savings of $3,363 over 4 years. This corresponds to a return on investment of $6.50 per dollar spent. This intervention yielded savings in every category of health care costs examined, including pharmacy, inpatient and outpatient medical, and mental health specialty care (Unützer et al. 2008). Similar cost savings have been identified in CC studies that included patients with depression and diabetes (Katon et al. 2008), patients with depression and multiple chronic medical conditions (Katon et al. 2012), and patients with severe anxiety (panic disorder) (Katon et al. 2002), as well as in medical CC programs for patients with serious mental illnesses (Druss et al. 2011). These findings from research studies are consistent with published data from large integrated health care systems, including Kaiser Permanente and Intermountain Healthcare, that have implemented CC programs and realized substantial cost savings associated with these programs (Grypma et al. 2006; Reiss-Brennan et al. 2010).

There are additional economic benefits from effective CC; depression substantially reduces productivity and effective workforce participation and lowers the chance that individuals who are unemployed will reenter the workforce (Katon 2009; Wang et al. 2008). Research shows that the systematic implementation of these programs for depression in primary care can reduce many of these negative economic effects of depression, resulting in improved personal income, employment (Schoenbaum et al. 2002; Wells et al. 2001), and other positive workplace outcomes (Wang et al. 2007).

In summary, the effectiveness and cost-effectiveness of CC have been established by more than 79 randomized controlled trials; CC is an outstanding example of an approach that helps achieve the "triple aim" in health care: improved patient care experiences, better health outcomes for populations, and lower health care costs.

CORE PRINCIPLES OF COLLABORATIVE CARE

A national expert panel convened by the Advancing Integrated Mental Health Solutions (AIMS) Center at the University of Washington identified five core principles of effective CC programs (http://aims.uw.edu/collaborative-care/principles-collaborative-care):

1. *Patient-centered care:* Primary care and behavioral health providers collaborate effectively on care teams using shared care plans.
2. *Evidence-based care:* Patients are offered treatments for which there is credible research evidence to support their efficacy in treating the target condition.
3. *Measurement-based treatment to target:* Each patient's care plan clearly articulates personal goals and clinical outcomes that are routinely measured. Treatments are adjusted if patients are not improving as expected.
4. *Population-based care:* The care team shares a defined group of patients tracked in a registry to make sure those patients do not "fall through the cracks." Practices track and reach out to patients who are not improving, and psychiatric consultants provide caseload-focused consultation on all patients who are not improving, not just ad hoc advice on select patients.
5. *Accountable care:* Providers are accountable and reimbursed for quality care and outcomes.

COLLABORATIVE CARE TEAM

To help implement such programs, psychiatrists typically work as part of a collaborative team that supports patients and their PCPs. Specific team members include the following:

- A patient who is actively participating in his or her care and responsible for working with the PCP and care manager (CM) to achieve goals set in a care plan and tracking clinical progress using a simple checklist such as a Patient Health Questionnaire depression rating scale (PHQ-9)
- A PCP, usually a family physician, internist, pediatrician, nurse-practitioner, or physician assistant, who makes an initial diagnosis and initiates treatment, often psychopharmacological treatment or referral for behavioral health counseling
- A CM (in some organizations also called a behavioral health provider or behavioral health consultant), such as a nurse, clinical social worker, or psychologist, who is based in primary care and trained to provide evidence-based care coordination, diagnostic assessments, brief behavioral interventions, and support of the treatments such as medications initiated by the PCP. In some cases, the CM is trained to provide evidence-based, brief/structured psychotherapy, such as cognitive-behavioral therapy or problem-solving treatment in primary care. In other cases, a CM may refer to other behavioral health professionals based in the practice or outside the practice for such evidence-based psychotherapies.

- A psychiatric consultant, usually a psychiatrist but possibly a nurse-practitioner or physician assistant certified in psychiatry, who advises the primary care treatment team with a focus on the subset of patients who present diagnostic challenges or who are not showing clinical improvements. Such consultation can be provided in person or through the use of telemedicine (telephonic or televideo consultation).

Psychiatric consultants on such teams typically provide a range of services that include 1) informal "curbside consultations" to CMs and PCPs in person or by telephone, 2) systematic case review meetings in which psychiatrists meet with a primary care–based CM and/or PCP to systematically review all patients on a clinician's panel who are presenting diagnostic or therapeutic challenges, and 3) occasional face-to-face consultations where they are requested by a PCP to see a patient in person or by televideo connection. Such face-to-face consultations are often focused on patients who present particular diagnostic or therapeutic challenges and who are not improving with existing treatment in primary care. Psychiatric consultants may convey treatment recommendations directly to the treating PCP or through a CM.

In terms of the clinical approach, CC programs follow the principles of measurement-based care (Trivedi 2009), treatment-to-target care, and stepped care (Von Korff and Tiemens 2000), and other aspects of the chronic illness care model proposed by Wagner et al. (1996). Each patient's progress is closely tracked using validated clinical rating scales (e.g., PHQ-9 [Kroenke et al. 2001]), analogous to how patients with diabetes are monitored by testing HbA1c levels. Treatment is systematically adjusted if patients are not improving as expected. Initial adjustments can be made by the primary care treatment team, with input from the psychiatric consultant if needed. Patients who continue not to respond to treatment or have an acute crisis are referred to behavioral health specialty care, as are patients who seek such referral. Such systematic "treatment to target" can overcome the "clinical inertia" that is often responsible for ineffective treatments of common mental disorders in primary care (Henke et al. 2009).

In the TEAMcare model, additional clinical oversight is provided by consulting PCPs (usually not the patient's treating PCP) to ensure medical disease targets are being met in addition to those for depression. Regular caseload review with the CMs is provided by the consultant PCP in addition to the consultant psychiatric provider, who work side by side in this model to improve both medical and behavioral health outcomes (Katon et al. 2010).

In summary, CC follows principles of good chronic illness management. It enhances usual primary care by adding three crucial services: 1) care coordination and care management for patients; 2) proactive monitoring and treatment to target using validated clinical rating scales; and 3) regular, systematic psychiatric caseload reviews and consultation for patients who do not show clinical improvement.

EXAMPLE PROGRAMS

CC has been successfully implemented in a number of health care organizations and health plans throughout the United States. These include state-wide implementations both with commercially insured adults, with urban and rural low-income safety net populations, and system-wide programs initiated by the Veterans Health Administration and Department of Defense. Several large health care organizations have undertaken large-scale implementations of this evidence-based program. These include national and regional health plans, including Kaiser Permanente and Intermountain Health (Grypma et al. 2006; Reiss-Brennan et al. 2010). In Minnesota, the Institute for Clinical System Improvement's Depression Improvement Across Minnesota, Offering a New Direction (DIAMOND) program (https://www.icsi.org/health_initiatives/mental_health/diamond_for_depression/) has implemented CC in partnership with 6 commercial health plans, 25 medical groups, and more than 80 primary care clinics across the state (Korsen and Pietruszewski 2009). Other large-scale implementations include the army's Re-engineering Systems of Primary Care Treatment in the Military (RESPECT-Mil) program (www.pdhealth.mil/respect-mil/index.asp), implemented in over 100 army primary care clinics in the United States and abroad, and the Department of Veterans Affairs' Veterans Health Administration (www.hsrd.research.va.gov/publications/internal/depression_primer.pdf), which has implemented it in hundreds of primary care clinics across the United States.

In the state of Washington, the Mental Health Integration Program (http://integratedcare-nw.org), which is jointly sponsored by the Community Health Plan of Washington and Public Health of Seattle and King County, has partnered with the AIMS Center at the University of Washington to integrate CC into over 140 community health clinics throughout the state, serving safety net patients with medical and behavioral health needs (Unützer et al. 2012). A group of 20 consulting psychiatrists (approximately 5 full-time equivalents) provide weekly caseload reviews of patients with the CMs in the participating primary care clinics, with quality of care and outcomes routinely tracked on a Web-based electronic registry. Over 35,000 patients have received care in this program, and an early evaluation has demonstrated beneficial effects in terms of reducing homelessness and arrest rates in this vulnerable population, in addition to high rates of engagement and improved quality of behavioral health care. Clinical outcomes are tracked on both individual and aggregate bases, and a recent study shows that clinical outcomes can be further improved when 25% of the payment for services is tied to clinics achieving specific quality performance measures (Unützer et al. 2012).

PAYMENT FOR COLLABORATIVE CARE

Payment for services has been identified as one of the barriers to the implementation of evidence-based CC programs (Butler et al. 2008). Large-scale implementations use a number of different payment approaches, ranging from fully capitated payment (e.g., Kaiser Permanente, Veterans Health Administration, Department of Defense) to case-rate payments (e.g., in Minnesota's DIAMOND program) that cover the costs of CMs and consulting psychiatrists. In the Washington Mental Health Integration Program, a health plan provides direct payments for the psychiatric caseload reviews and consultations based on the number of clinics, caseloads, and CMs supported by the psychiatric consultant. Additional approaches to payment for CC are being tested nationally through funding from the Patient Protection and Affordable Care Act and the Center for Medicare & Medicaid Innovation (http://innovation.cms.gov). Traditional fee-for-service payment arrangements do not yet pay for psychiatric consultation and case reviews that do not involve direct patient contact, but several health care systems pay for such services in a way similar to how they cover liaison psychiatry services. This kind of systematic caseload-focused psychiatric consultation may become increasingly relevant as health care organizations develop patient-centered medical homes and accountable care organizations that are charged with providing comprehensive care for defined populations of patients, who often have limited access to or use of traditional mental health services, while containing overall health care costs.

CONCLUSION

Collaborative care creates important opportunities for psychiatrists to help achieve the triple aim of health care reform: 1) to improve the patient care experience, 2) to improve the health of populations, and 3) to reduce the cost of health care. The strong research evidence for the effectiveness and cost-effectiveness of CC, along with robust experience implementing such programs in diverse health care systems around the country, suggests that public and private payers will increasingly turn to psychiatrists to help implement and provide such services. For psychiatrists, this presents a new way to practice as part of a team, meeting the medical and behavioral health needs of large patient populations and developing satisfying and rewarding relationships not only with patients but also with other team members. Such teamwork also presents important opportunities for psychiatrists to share their unique expertise with other colleagues such as CMs, PCPs, and other behavioral health specialists.

REFERENCES

Archer J, Bower P, Gilbody S, et al: Collaborative care for depression and anxiety problems. Cochrane Database of Systematic Reviews 2012, Issue 10. Art. No.: CD006525. DOI: 10.1002/14651858.CD006525.pub2.

Arean PA, Ayalon L, Hunkeler E, et al: Improving depression care for older, minority patients in primary care. Med Care 43(4):381–390, 2005

Bogner HR, Morales KH, De Vries HF, et al: Integrated management of type 2 diabetes mellitus and depression treatment to improve medication adherence: a randomized controlled trial. Ann Fam Med 10(1):15–22, 2012

Butler M, Kane RL, McAlpine D, et al: Integration of mental health/substance abuse and primary care. Evid Rep Technol Assess 173:1–362, 2008

Community Preventive Services Task Force: Recommendation from the Community Preventive Services Task Force for use of collaborative care for the management of depressive disorders. Am J Prev Med 42(5):521–524, 2012

Cunningham PJ: Beyond parity: primary care physicians' perspectives on access to mental health care. Health Aff (Millwood) 28(3):490–501, 2009

Druss BG, Von Esenwein SA, Compton MT, et al: Budget impact and sustainability of medical care management for persons with serious mental illnesses. Am J Psychiatry 168(11):1171–1178, 2011

Ell K, Katon W, Cabassa LJ, et al: Depression and diabetes among low-income Hispanics: design elements of a socioculturally adapted collaborative care model randomized controlled trial. Int J Psychiatry Med 39(2):113–132, 2009

Ell K, Aranda MP, Xie B, et al: Collaborative depression treatment in older and younger adults with physical illness: pooled comparative analysis of three randomized clinical trials. Am J Geriatr Psychiatry 18(6):520–530, 2010a

Ell K, Katon W, Xie B, et al: Collaborative care management of major depression among low-income, predominantly Hispanic subjects with diabetes: a randomized controlled trial. Diabetes Care 33(4):706–713, 2010b

Gilbody S, Bower P, Fletcher J, et al: Collaborative care for depression: a cumulative meta-analysis and review of longer-term outcomes. Arch Intern Med 166(21):2314–2321, 2006a

Gilbody S, Bower P, Whitty P: Costs and consequences of enhanced primary care for depression: systematic review of randomised economic evaluations. Br J Psychiatry 189:297–308, 2006b

Glied S, Herzog K, Frank R: Review: the net benefits of depression management in primary care. Med Care Res Rev 67(3):251–274, 2010

Grembowski DE, Martin D, Patrick DL, et al: Managed care, access to mental health specialists, and outcomes among primary care patients with depressive symptoms. J Gen Intern Med 17(4):258–269, 2002

Grypma L, Haverkamp R, Little S, et al: Taking an evidence-based model of depression care from research to practice: making lemonade out of depression. Gen Hosp Psychiatry 28(2):101–107, 2006

Henke RM, Zaslavsky AM, McGuire TG, et al: Clinical inertia in depression treatment. Med Care 47(9):959–967, 2009

Katon WJ: Clinical and health services relationships between major depression, depressive symptoms, and general medical illness. Biol Psychiatry 54(3):216–226, 2003

Katon WJ: The impact of depression on workplace functioning and disability costs. Am J Manag Care 15 (11 suppl):S322–S327, 2009

Katon WJ, Unützer J: Health reform and the Affordable Care Act: the importance of mental health treatment to achieving the triple aim. J Psychosom Res 74(6):533–537, 2013

Katon WJ, Roy-Byrne P, Russo J, et al: Cost-effectiveness and cost offset of a collaborative care intervention for primary care patients with panic disorder. Arch Gen Psychiatry 59(12):1098–1104, 2002

Katon WJ, Lin E, Russo J, et al: Increased medical costs of a population-based sample of depressed elderly patients. Arch Gen Psychiatry 60(9):897–903, 2003

Katon WJ, Russo JE, Von Korff M, et al: Long-term effects on medical costs of improving depression outcomes in patients with depression and diabetes. Diabetes Care 31(6):1155–1159, 2008

Katon WJ, Lin EH, Von Korff M, et al: Collaborative care for patients with depression and chronic illnesses. N Engl J Med 363(27):2611–2620, 2010

Katon WJ, Russo J, Lin EH, et al: Cost-effectiveness of a multicondition collaborative care intervention: a randomized controlled trial. Arch Gen Psychiatry 69(5):506–514, 2012

Korsen N, Pietruszewski P: Translating evidence to practice: two stories from the field. J Clin Psychol Med Settings 16(1):47–57, 2009

Kroenke K, Spitzer RL, Williams JB: The PHQ-9: validity of a brief depression severity measure. J Gen Intern Med 16(9):606–613, 2001

Levine SL, Unützer J, Yip JY, et al: Physicians' satisfaction with a collaborative disease management program for late-life depression in primary care. Gen Hosp Psychiatry 27:383–391, 2005

Miranda J, Duan N, Sherbourne C, et al: Improving care for minorities: can quality improvement interventions improve care and outcomes for depressed minorities? Results of a randomized, controlled trial. Health Serv Res 38(2):613–630, 2003

Miranda J, Schoenbaum M, Sherbourne C, et al: Effects of primary care depression treatment on minority patients' clinical status and employment. Arch Gen Psychiatry 61(8):827–834, 2004

Moussavi S, Chatterji S, Verdes E, et al: Depression, chronic diseases, and decrements in health: results from the World Health Surveys. Lancet 370(9590):851–858, 2007

National Committee for Quality Assurance: Standards for Patient-Centered Medical Home Care. Washington, DC, National Committee for Quality Assurance, 2011

Patel V, Belkin GS, Chockalingam A, et al: Grand challenges: integrating mental health services into priority health care platforms. PLoS Med 10(5):e1001448, 2013

Regier DA, Narrow WE, Rae DS, et al: The de facto US mental and addictive disorders service system. Epidemiologic Catchment Area prospective 1-year prevalence rates of disorders and services. Arch Gen Psychiatry 50(2):85–94, 1993

Reilly S, Planner C, Gask L, et al: Collaborative care approaches for people with severe mental illness. Cochrane Database of Systematic Reviews 2013, Issue 11. Art. No.: CD009531. DOI: 10.1002/14651858.CD009531.pub2.

Reiss-Brennan B, Briot PC, Savitz LA, et al: Cost and quality impact of Intermountain's mental health integration program. J Healthc Manag 55(2):97–113, 2010

Roy-Byrne PP, Craske MG, Stein MB, et al: A randomized effectiveness trial of cognitive-behavioral therapy and medication for primary care panic disorder. Arch Gen Psychiatry 62(3):290–298, 2005

Rush AJ, Trivedi M, Carmody TJ, et al: One-year clinical outcomes of depressed public sector outpatients: a benchmark for subsequent studies. Biol Psychiatry 56(1):46–53, 2004

Schoenbaum M, Unützer J, McCaffrey D, et al: The effects of primary care depression treatment on patients' clinical status and employment. Health Serv Res 37(5):1145–1158, 2002

Simon G: Collaborative care for mood disorders. Curr Opin Psychiatry 22(1):37–41, 2009

Simon GE, VonKorff M, Barlow W: Health care costs of primary care patients with recognized depression. Arch Gen Psychiatry 52(10):850–856, 1995

Simon GE, Ding V, Hubbard R, et al: Early dropout from psychotherapy for depression with group- and network-model therapists. Adm Policy Ment Health 39(6):440–447, 2012

Stewart JC, Perkins AJ, Callahan CM: Effect of collaborative care for depression on risk of cardiovascular events: data from the IMPACT randomized controlled trial. Psychosom Med 76(1):29-37, 2014

Thota AB, Sipe TA, Byard GJ, et al: Collaborative care to improve the management of depressive disorders: a Community Guide systematic review and meta-analysis. Am J Prev Med 42(5):525–538, 2012

Trivedi MH: Treating depression to full remission. J Clin Psychiatry 70(1):e01, 2009

Uebelacker LA, Smith M, Lewis AW, et al: Treatment of depression in a low-income primary care setting with colocated mental health care. Fam Syst Health 27(2):161–171, 2009

Unützer J, Patrick DL, Simon G, et al: Depressive symptoms and the cost of health services in HMO patients aged 65 years and older: a 4-year prospective study. JAMA 277(20):1618–1623, 1997

Unützer J, Katon W, Callahan CM, et al: Collaborative-care management of late-life depression in the primary care setting. JAMA 288(22):2836–2845, 2002

Unützer J, Katon WJ, Fan MY, et al: Long-term cost effects of collaborative care for late-life depression. Am J Manag Care 14(2):95–100, 2008

Unützer J, Chan YF, Hafer E, et al: Quality improvement with pay-for-performance incentives in integrated behavioral health care. Am J Public Health 102(6):e41–45, 2012

U.S. Department of Health and Human Services: Mental Health: A Report of the Surgeon General. Rockville, MD, U.S. Department of Health and Human Services, Substance Abuse and Mental Health Services Administration, Center for Mental Health Services, National Institutes of Health, National Institute of Mental Health, 1999. Available at: www.surgeongeneral.gov/library/mentalhealth/home.html

Von Korff M, Tiemens B: Individualized stepped care of chronic illness. West J Med 172(2):133–137, 2000

Wagner EH, Austin BT, Von Korff M: Organizing care for patients with chronic illness. Milbank Q 74(4):511–544, 1996

Wang PS, Lane M, Olfson M, et al: Twelve-month use of mental health services in the United States: results from the National Comorbidity Survey Replication. Arch Gen Psychiatry 62(6):629–640, 2005

Wang PS, Demler O, Olfson M, et al: Changing profiles of service sectors used for mental health care in the United States. Am J Psychiatry 163(7):1187–1198, 2006

Wang PS, Simon GE, Avorn J, et al: Telephone screening, outreach, and care management for depressed workers and impact on clinical and work productivity outcomes: a randomized controlled trial. JAMA 298(12):1401–1411, 2007

Wang PS, Simon GE, Kessler RC: Making the business case for enhanced depression care: the National Institute of Mental Health-Harvard Work Outcomes Research and Cost-effectiveness Study. J Occup Environ Med 50(4):468–475, 2008

Wells K, Klap R, Koike A, et al: Ethnic disparities in unmet need for alcoholism, drug abuse, and mental health care. Am J Psychiatry 158(12):2027–2032, 2001

Woltmann E, Grogan-Kaylor A, Perron B, et al: Comparative effectiveness of collaborative chronic care models for mental health conditions across primary, specialty, and behavioral health care settings: systematic review and meta-analysis. Am J Psychiatry 169(8):790–804, 2012

CHAPTER 2

The Collaborative Care Team in Action

Lori Raney, M.D.

Gina Lasky, Ph.D.

Clare Scott, LCSW

The core principles of effective collaborative care (CC) were introduced in Chapter 1 ("Evidence Base and Core Principles"): 1) patient-centered care, 2) evidence-based care, 3) measurement-based treatment to target, 4) population-based care, and 5) accountable care, and they serve as a guide for determining the essential ingredients of these integrated programs. The mnemonic TEMP-A (for team-based, evidence-based, measurement-based, population-based, and accountable) can be helpful in remembering the core principles and serve as a compass to guide development and successful implementation of collaborative care. This chapter will demonstrate how these principles are put into action in the primary care setting, while adding at least two new team members to the traditional primary care lineup: a care manager or behavioral health provider (BHP) and a consulting psychiatric provider. The tasks of these new team members will be more fully described later; however, their presence enables the primary care team to better recognize and adequately treat the behavioral health conditions that have historically been overlooked and inadequately treated in primary care settings. This enhanced team can provide immediate access to behavioral health treatment and reach a greater population of patients, which can lead to a significant (positive) impact on public health.

CULTURE OF PRIMARY CARE

The primary care environment is quite different from what professionals working in behavioral health are accustomed to and is marked by the rapid cadence of care and the wide range of health care issues presenting for the primary care providers (PCPs) to manage. In the primary care setting, treatment is traditionally physician driven, and the team supports the PCP in their management of the patient. The focus is often on conditions that present with the highest acuity at that visit, which may leave little time to address other issues or attempt to discover underlying contributions to the presenting problems. PCPs tend to have large panels of patients that present episodically for care, and charts are not typically "closed" as occurs in behavioral health settings. PCPs and BHPs often view the same patients through different lenses (and language), and these dissimilarities can lead to misunderstandings at times in the primary care setting. Some examples of these differences are listed in Table 2–1.

TABLE 2–1.   Differences between primary care and behavioral health cultures

Primary care environment	Behavioral health environment
Flexible boundaries	Firm boundaries
Empathy, compassion	Professional distance, neutrality
Open access and communication	Mutual accountability
Shifting roles	Consistent roles
Flexible schedule	Fixed schedule
Continuity over time	Treat and "close the chart," "terminate care"
Use of clinical guidelines	Individual treatment planning
Data shared between providers	Data private and "confidential"
Treatment dependent on external data (laboratory results, X-ray)	Treatment embodied in the relationship with provider
Disease management	Recovery model and meaningful lives
"Fix it"	Assist in the change process

Example of Cultural Differences Between a Primary Care Provider and Behavioral Health Provider

This all makes me remember the discussions I have had with our behavioral specialist in our office. My boundaries to patients, life, and work are very much looser than hers. She works far fewer hours, does not see patients with certain problems, will only see patients that pay her, and the list goes on. I have looked at this with questions over the past 2 years: questions about commitment, caring, job understanding, "How can we help by saying NO so much." She would say "Saying NO is as important as saying YES." The reflection at the moment is thinking about all the MDs I know—most are angry/tired/burnt out. The therapists I know are relaxed and happy. Maybe we MDs have a lot to learn from the behavioral health providers?

G.K., PCP, Colorado

CORE TASKS AND COMPONENTS

The CC team engages in a work flow that consists of specific steps to meet the intent of the core principles (TEMP-A). These steps are to *screen, treat, track,* and *feed back* the results to the care team to make adjustments as needed. Each of these tasks will be described in detail.

Screening

The first task of the team, and an important element of population-based care, is to identify patients who may have behavioral health needs in addition to the physical health symptoms that led to the appointment. Behavioral health needs may be stated in a patient's chief complaint, arise during the appointment with the PCP, or be uncovered through a detection process known as *population-based screening,* where patients seen for care in the clinic are given a core set of screening measures. This screening could include all patients coming to the clinic for any reason or could be targeted toward a select group such as pregnant women or patients with a diagnosis of diabetes. Utilizing tools to identify symptoms of psychosocial distress notifies the team of potential issues so that further evaluation can occur. Key tools that identify symptoms of depression, anxiety, and substance use disorders, the most common mental disorders found in primary care settings (Olfson et al. 1997), can lead to detection of these illnesses. These screening tools are not unlike the traditional vital signs taken at the onset of most primary care visits, which are utilized to discern abnormalities in temperature, weight, blood pressure, pulse, and respirations. Together, these two categories of screening allow for a set of *comprehensive* vital signs to help guide the next step of the primary care visit, providing an all-inclusive, whole-person approach to the care. Table 2-2 shows a person whose vital signs indicate high blood pressure, excessive weight, depression, and alcohol use that need further investigation.

TABLE 2–2. Comprehensive vital signs

Temperature	98.6
Pulse	75
Respirations	12
Blood pressure	**140/95**
Body mass index	**27**
PHQ-9	**16**
GAD-7	5
AUDIT	**10**
PC-PTSD-	0

Note.   AUDIT = Alcohol Use Disorders Identification Test; GAD = Generalized Anxiety Disorder Scale; PC-PTSD = Primary Care PTSD Screen; PHQ-9 = Patient Health Questionnaire depression rating scale. Boldface values show elevated blood pressure and body mass index in addition to a high score on the PHQ screen for depression and the AUDIT screening tool for alcohol use.

Common "front office" screening tools utilized in primary care include the Patient Health Questionnaire depression rating scale (PHQ-9; Kroenig and Spitzer 2001), the seven-item Generalized Anxiety Disorder Scale (GAD-7; Spitzer et al. 2006), and the Alcohol Use Disorders Identification Test (AUDIT; Saunders et al. 1993). Screening can also include other tools, like the Primary Care PTSD Screen (PC-PTSD; Prins et al. 2003) and the Drug Abuse Screening Test (DAST; Gavin et al. 1989) for illicit drug use. Additional "back office" screens such as the Mood Disorders Questionnaire (MDQ; Hirschfeld et al. 2000) and tests of cognition such as the Mini-Mental State Examination (MMSE; Folstein et al. 1975) can be completed later in the appointment if additional information is needed to clarify the diagnosis. Sometimes shorter versions of these tools are used, such as the PHQ-2, the GAD-2, and the AUDIT-C, which allow fewer questions to be asked initially and if positive can lead to more complete evaluation if needed. However, some of these screening tools are also used in tracking improvement (PHQ-9 and GAD-7), and using the shorter version can confuse the data-gathering process when the numbers do not directly correlate with the longer forms. These tools can be administered in a variety of ways, including on paper by the patient in the waiting room, verbally with direct entry into an electronic health record, on electronic tablets or other handheld devices, in waiting room kiosks, online, and by phone prior to or between visits depending on how an organization decides to position them in the work flow. Frequency of screening is often every 6 months to yearly if results are negative and for those tools that are also used for tracking response to treatment (such as PHQ-9 and GAD-7) at each visit if initially positive until a targeted end point is reached (e.g., PHQ-9 <5). Table 2–3 lists some of the common screening tools utilized in primary care and the usual cutoffs, and Table 2–4 is the PHQ-9, one of the most frequently used assessment tools in clinical practice and research. It is important to remember these are screening tools and making a firm diagnosis requires additional history gathering for confirmation of a diagnosis.

TABLE 2–3. Commonly used screening tools in primary care settings

Mood disorders	Anxiety disorders	Psychotic disorders	Substance use disorders	Cognitive disorders
PHQ-9— depression (>9 or positive on #9 suicidal thoughts)	GAD-7— anxiety (>7)	BPRS— psychotic symptoms	AUDIT— alcohol use (>7 for women and >8 for men)	Mini-Mental State Examination (>14)
MDQ—bipolar disorder	PC-PTSD— PTSD	Positive and Negative Syndrome Scale	CAGE— alcohol use	Mini Cog
CIDI—bipolar disorder	Young Brown— OCD		DAST— drug use	Montreal Cognitive Assessment

Note. AUDIT = Alcohol Use Disorders Identification Test; BPRS = Brief Psychiatric Rating Scale; CIDI = Composite International Diagnostic Interview; DAST = Drug Abuse Screening Test; GAD-7 = seven-item Generalized Anxiety Disorder Scale; MDQ = Mood Disorder Questionnaire; OCD = obsessive-compulsive disorder; PC-PTSD = Primary Care PTSD Screen; PHQ-9, Patient Health Questionnaire depression rating scale.

Treatment

Once a behavioral health issue is identified through screening or self-report, the next step is to engage patients in the collaborative treatment process. Ide-

TABLE 2–4.   Patient Health Questionnaire-9 (PHQ-9)

Name _____   Date _____

Over the last 2 weeks, how long have you been bothered by any of the following?	Not at all	Several days	More than half the days	Nearly every day
1. Little interest or pleasure in doing things	0	1	2	3
2. Feeling down, depressed, or hopeless	0	1	2	3
3. Trouble falling or staying asleep or sleeping too much	0	1	2	3
4. Feeling tired or having little energy	0	1	2	3
5. Poor appetite or overeating	0	1	2	3
6. Feeling bad about yourself—or that you are a failure or have let yourself or your family down	0	1	2	3
7. Trouble concentrating on things, such as reading the newspaper or watching television	0	1	2	3
8. Moving or speaking so slowly that other people could have noticed. Or the opposite—being so fidgety or restless that you have been moving around a lot more than usual	0	1	2	3
9. Thoughts that you would be better off dead or of hurting yourself in some way	0	1	2	3
Total score of all four columns				

If you checked off *any* problems, how *difficult* have these problems made it for you to do your work, take care of things at home, or get along with other people?

❏ Not difficult at all   ❏ Somewhat difficult   ❏ Very difficult   ❏ Extremely difficult

Source.   Pfizer Inc., available at www.phqscreeners.com.

ally, the treatment philosophy in the clinic has been explained ahead of the appointment through the use of educational and promotional tools to notify patients that the clinic is dedicated to providing whole-person care, which includes psychological well-being in addition to physical health. The screening results can be utilized by a variety of personnel, including a receptionist or a medical assistant or a nurse who takes vital signs and rooms the patient. Depending on the level of staff autonomy allowed, any of these staff members could begin the process of preparing the patient for the next steps. This could include "flagging" a room for BHP intervention prior to the PCP arrival, which could lead to the BHP going into the exam room, introducing himself or herself to the patient, and explaining his or her role on the team. This can also be utilized when the PCP is behind schedule by making use of the time the patient is in the room waiting to begin the behavioral health assessment. It could also include a process called a "warm handoff," where the PCP starts the appointment with the patient, realizes the need for BHP assistance, and then proceeds to introduce the patient to the BHP during the course of the exam. The BHP is introduced as a "member of the health care team" and usually not initially as a therapist. The goal is to normalize the experience of having the BHP intervene by using language that avoids compartmentalizing the care into a separate behavioral health category to reduce the stigma that sometimes accompanies behavioral health treatment and the resistance that often follows.

The next steps in the integrated setting follow a system known as "stepped care" (Von Korff and Tiemens 2000), which allows effective treatment to be provided with just the resources necessary at that level. The person receives the care he or she needs without overutilization of resources, leading to improved outcomes that are cost-efficient. The first rung on the stepped-care ladder is *self-management,* in which the patient is handling his or her health care on his or her own outside the primary care setting. This includes the use of diet, exercise, education, stress management techniques, and/or family and community supports to cope with any health conditions or stressors he or she is experiencing. On the second rung, the patient *discusses his or her concerns with his or her PCP only* without involving other staff. For example, the PCP may review the results of a PHQ-9 that was slightly elevated and decide to increase an existing antidepressant without the need for additional team member assistance. Treatment at the third rung of the stepped-care ladder now engages the *assistance of the BHP* and can occur proactively in a clinic where a staff member (e.g., medical assistant, nurse, receptionist) notifies the BHP of a concern or the PCP directly requests assistance. The need could be for diagnostic clarification or provision of a brief therapeutic intervention at the time of the appointment and could involve a warm handoff accompanied by scheduling an appointment at a later date. At the fourth rung, the *psychiatrist has been engaged* to provide consultation to the team, often for diagnostic clarification or medication recommendation, allowing the treatment to move forward without delay. While the majority of the time the psychiatric consultation is handled by phone, in some instances direct evaluation of the patient by the consultant psychiatrist is necessary and can be arranged in person or by televideo, moving up another step in the process. Further rungs up the stepped-care ladder involve utilization of external *specialty behavioral health services* (e.g., group therapy such as dialectical behavior therapy) and may sometimes proceed to *inpatient hospitalization.* When the team is functioning well, treatment is provided at the intensity needed at any given visit and will not have to progress through these steps if a higher level of intervention is not warranted. For instance, someone who is actively suicidal can be immediately referred to inpatient psychiatric care if that is the recommended treatment at that visit, bypassing all the other levels of care.

Once introduced to the patient as a member of the care team, the BHP does a brief diagnostic assessment, utilizing information already gathered by the PCP, the screening tools, and the medical record. The job is to quickly assess the situation and determine what additional interventions are needed. This may include diagnostic clarification that leads the PCP to begin a medication trial and a brief intervention such as behavioral activation (discussed in section "Collaborative Care Team") and may include a call to the psychiatrist for medication consultation if needed. Another important aspect of the job is assessing the individual for any additional referrals that may be useful, such as support groups, individual therapy, or community resources. Follow-up appointments are scheduled, and the treatment is documented in the patient record. Figure 2–1 illustrates the workings of the team.

Rural settings often present challenges in recruiting and hiring the BHP and psychiatric consultant staff for this model. Research in utilizing telemedicine-based communication is under way, and at least one study (Fortney et al. 2013) has demonstrated the effectiveness of using an off-site team for the BHP and psychiatric consultation. Patient engagement with a BHP who communicates by telephone rather than being introduced via a warm handoff may be challenging and could present a barrier to successful implementation. Persistence in forming a mutually acceptable form of communication will be necessary as well as developing an understanding that some patients may simply choose not to engage.

Tracking

An important core feature and principle of population-based care is the use of an organizing tool, or registry, to track patient progress so changes can be made if improvement is not occurring and patients who are not engaging in treatment can be identified for follow-up. A registry contains data about a

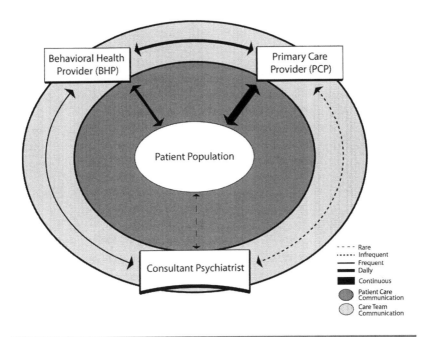

FIGURE 2–1. Collaborative care team communication.
Source. © Collaborative Care Consulting. Courtesy Dr. Lori Raney.

group of patients, such as baseline and most recent PHQ-9 scores, that allow the providers to follow an individual's progress and the group's aggregate response to treatment. In electronic registries, data points such as PHQ-9 scores can be sorted highest to lowest if desired to see who may have the greatest need for intervention and to allow the team to focus on the group that is not improving (Table 2–5). In this model, the BHP and psychiatric provider meet on a regular basis to review the caseload and determine if adjustments need to be made, including medication changes, diagnostic clarification, referrals for other types of treatment, changes in brief therapeutic interventions, and scheduling a direct (face-to-face) evaluation with the consulting psychiatrist. Once this measurement-based, treat-to-target approach has been used and a patient reaches his or her goal, relapse prevention planning takes place and the patient moves back into the routine maintenance and screening cycle.

Program Review and Feedback

Regular meetings to review outcomes for targeting areas for improvement and to adjust treatment approaches are a key process for the CC team and an important aspect of quality improvement. Following the progression of

TABLE 2–5. Prioritizing patients to be reviewed utilizing registry data for depression

Patient	Enrollment date	PHQ BL	Date last seen	PHQ-9 most recent	Recommendations
A	3/11/2013	22	5/22/2013	**24**	Refer for direct evaluation
B	2/24/2013	18	4/18/2013	**18**	Refer to DBT
C	3/1/2013	23	4/22/2013	17	Increase antidepressant
D	2/11/2013	15	4/7/2013	13	Refer to SA counseling
E	4/2/2013	21	5/9/2013	12	Give current medications more time
F	2/1/2013	16	5/20/2013	6	No changes
G	1/15/2013	20	5/18/2013	3	Relapse prevention plan

Note. BL = baseline; DBT = dialectical behavior therapy; PHQ-9 = Patient Health Questionnaire depression rating scale; PSA = substance abuse. Values in boldface indicate elevated scores and are the patients who would be prioritized for discussion.

screening, treating, and tracking mentioned above, this last step is to provide feedback to the care team. Utilizing aggregate data from the registry allows the team to identify gaps in care that may signify the need for additional training or discover areas where interventions have been successful and warrant expansion. For example, the team notices in reviewing the registry that patients with both chronic pain and depression are not improving as quickly as desired. As a result, the team decides additional training in therapeutic and medication interventions for chronic pain is needed to see if this can lead to better outcomes. Another example is the team noticing one BHP is showing more rapid improvement in reaching targeted outcomes on the PHQ-9 than the other BHPs on the team; the team then works to discover if there is a special technique being utilized that others can implement. In the TEAMcare model (Katon et al. 2010), side-by-side tracking of both measurements of depression and other health parameters such as blood pressure can demonstrate to PCPs and others that treating depression can have additional health benefits. In addition, statistics from the registry can be used to show the value of the model and help demonstrate the effectiveness of CC for those who may be skeptical about its efficacy or have administrative oversight, including board members of organizations. These kinds of data can prove how a clinic can be accountable for the care provided and may one day be used to determine reimbursement structures, payment for outcomes, and models that help reach the triple aim in health care (see Chapter 1, "Evidence Base and Core Principles").

COLLABORATIVE CARE TEAM

Behavioral Health Providers

BHPs, referred to in some systems as behavioral health consultants or care managers, are mainly trained in social work, psychology, and nursing and provide a wide array of behavioral health interventions across a range of diagnoses. Individuals who are a good fit for this job enjoy the fast-paced cadence of care seen in the primary care setting and the ever-changing demands that present over the course of the day. BHPs need to be flexible, creative, and self-confident and enjoy working as a member of a team. The willingness to be interrupted is crucial to the flow when PCPs find themselves in situations that need immediate consultation to provide effective treatment and avoid unnecessary referral. The ability to listen to and quickly engage a patient is a skill that is invaluable and often takes time to perfect.

Therapists who are used to and enjoy long-term relationships with patients in hour-long sessions may not be suited for the BHP role unless they are excited about making significant changes in the way they practice and are able to adapt to the needs and culture of primary care. This is a major paradigm shift that should not be underestimated in staff that is often moving out of traditional roles to join CC teams as BHPs. It is very important to this model that the BHP does not inadvertently engage in a more colocated psychotherapy (i.e., simple referral from PCP to the BHP, who then provides traditional hour-long therapy sessions) because this prevents ready access and consultation as the caseload grows and waiting times increase. A good fit for the BHP role is often a therapist who has worked in emergency or crisis service positions and understands the concepts of triage, the need to quickly shift gears, and inconsistency in the work flow.

The most effective BHPs also possess skills in rapid diagnostic assessment that usually come from several years in practice. The ability to gather information quickly and then efficiently recite it back in a concise presentation is important in the flow of the clinic setting, with rushed PCPs and a busy consultant psychiatrist on the phone, both of whom need to clearly understand the patient's presentation and status. Excellent communication skills and the tenacity and tact to state their opinions are both important to the success of BHPs. They will also have in their toolbox skills in delivering evidence-based brief interventions, including motivational interviewing, behavioral activation (BA), problem-solving therapy (PST), and distress tolerance skills, to name a few of the most used treatments (discussed in section "Evidence-Based Brief Interventions Overview"). In some settings, they may need to be competent to treat across the life span and provide consultation for adolescents and children, utilizing a different set of screening instruments and interventions (see Chapter 4, "Child and Adolescent Psychiatry in Integrated Settings"). BHPs are also asked to intervene in health behavior change, such as helping an individual who is obese and noncompliant with a diabetes regimen identify barriers to managing his or her illness. This could include providing education and guidance on other health issues such as sleep, diet, exercise, and medication compliance. Knowledge of common medical conditions can be helpful when working on health behavior change goals in patients with illnesses such as diabetes and hypertension. Working in clinics implementing the TEAMcare model (Katon et al. 2010) that addresses multiple chronic conditions, including diabetes, hypertension, and dyslipidemias along with depression, will require knowledge of both medical condition management and health behavior change approaches.

A BHP's transition to a care team requires specific behavior changes in order to function effectively. An innovative approach to supporting the required changes is the use of a shadowing tool. This is a list that has several functions: an observation tool, a descriptor of the specific expected behaviors, and a checklist (Table 2–6). The BHP in training observes and notes the actions and language used by a seasoned BHP. A similar tool can be adapted to any role on a care team.

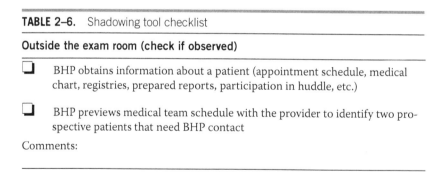

TABLE 2–6.   Shadowing tool checklist

Outside the exam room (check if observed)

❏   BHP obtains information about a patient (appointment schedule, medical chart, registries, prepared reports, participation in huddle, etc.)

❏   BHP previews medical team schedule with the provider to identify two prospective patients that need BHP contact

Comments:

With the move toward patient-centered medical homes and treating multiple chronic conditions, there may be a shift in determining the best staff configuration to serve in the BHP/care manager role(s). The skill sets of both nurses and behavioral health staff such as social workers and psychologists will be needed, and it will be prudent to remember the BHP's skills in rapid assessment and providing behavioral health interventions cannot be performed by just anyone on the team. It is the ability to quickly recognize a behavioral health condition that can lead to immediate and effective treatment in the primary care setting. This need to determine the best staffing configuration will most likely present a unique challenge over the next several years from the time of the writing of this chapter and will require careful consideration in the design of CC teams for the future.

The BHP often serves as a conveyor of information between the PCP and the consultant psychiatrist and is frequently called upon by the PCP to contact the psychiatrist for medication recommendations. Therefore, a certain level of trust needs to develop over time between these three team members to facilitate the flow of information. While initially the PCP may want to connect more directly with the psychiatric provider, there is typically a notable change over the course of the relationship where the PCP begins to trust the BHP's expertise and skills and how efficient the BHP can be in conveying information to and from the consultant psychiatrist. Conversely, the psychiatric provider must be able to rely on and trust the BHP's assessment of the patient and the BHP's ability to provide a sufficient case presentation in order to make recommendations. Establishing communication approaches that work for the members of the team is important, and a skillful BHP will work to find the best methods for each provider. These may include the use of e-mail, text messaging, mobile phone, televideo, or direct communication, depending on the preference of the PCP and psychiatric consultant. Understanding Health Insurance Portability and Accountability Act (HIPAA) regulations to allow effective and timely communication (e.g., if the BHP and PCP are from separate organizations) between team members is crucial and should not be mistakenly used as a barrier to communication (see more in Chapter 5, "Risk Management and Liability Issues in Integrated Care"). If a patient is not improving, the BHP is the gatekeeper for arranging a more intensive intervention, such as on-site or televideo direct evaluation of the patient by the consulting psychiatric provider. This is an important role because it prevents colocation of the psychiatrist by busy PCPs who may prefer to have a patient's behavioral health issues taken care of by a specialist and not go through the stepped-care process that allows this model to make the most efficient use of limited psychiatric resources.

Two Behavioral Health Provider Experiences

I enjoy the pace of practice, the logic of attaching the head to the body and destigmatizing behavioral health interventions.

BHP, CC practice, Colorado

Often the patients had a mixture of problems, and so it would be easy to get overwhelmed and feel like you have to create a plan to fix them all (traditional behavioral health). What I loved about the

BHP role was actually the simplicity of feeling like all I had to do was address the most important issue for that day. What we did (behavior activation or distress tolerance) may relate to any number of problems (depression, sleep, weight management, etc.), but it simplified the need for the moment. I think that having experience with diagnosis, risk assessment, and brief intervention does impact the BHP's ability to see both the big picture of diagnosis and assessment while narrowing in on the key skill for the day. The next microchange that will address much of the macropicture. I also think experience makes for a calm BHP, who is not pressured, anxious in front of a physician, or easily overwhelmed. They can flow with the situation more easily and demonstrate confidence and education for the physician and psychiatrist.

BHP, integrated practice, Colorado

Primary Care Providers

While clinics may have choices in the selection of well-versed BHP and psychiatric provider additions to their primary care team, it is often not possible to do this sort of preselection with the PCPs. Therefore, the work of educating, engaging, and modeling this system of care often falls to the BHP and psychiatric consultant. Experience has demonstrated a variety of responses when the CC model is proposed in primary care settings. Responses range from welcome relief for help with challenging and time-consuming patients, to a PCP who may believe the BHP will slow them down if they take time to address behavioral health issues, to a PCP asserting no need for additional help, believing adequate recognition and treatment of behavioral health conditions already occurs. Another frequent concern is that clinic-based population screening will uncover a host of problems that neither the current primary care system nor specialty behavioral health services, which PCPs have historically found unreliable for referrals, have the capacity to address. Upon learning the psychiatrist will not be conducting on-site examinations for all patients referred, many PCPs who do not yet understand the model will often voice frustration and skepticism. Working with patients in this model will be an uncomfortable experience initially for many PCPs as they adjust to having another team member taking part in the care of the patient. It may also take some time to demonstrate the model will not interfere with productivity and may actually improve efficiency because it allows the PCP to move on to his or her next patient while the BHP provides intervention and addresses the "puddle of tears." Many PCPs experience a sense of relief that someone else can "take the load off my plate," "speed me up," or "help buy me some time to finish my note" while the BHP is interacting with the patient. Reassurance can come with education about the model's effectiveness as seen in many of the meta-analyses presented in Chapter 1 and by showing the PCPs studies on clinician satisfaction with the CC model (Levine et al. 2005). Additional encouragement can also come from demonstrating the improvement in other health outcomes when behavioral health conditions are treated as shown in the TEAMcare trial, where HbA1c, low-density lipoprotein cholesterol, and blood pressure scores in patients with multiple chronic conditions decreased as the depression was treated (Katon et al. 2010). There are many excellent journal articles that can be shared with PCPs to help obtain buy-in and cooperation with CC implementation (see Chapter 1).

If acceptance and engagement in the process are not forthcoming, the BHP and psychiatrist can work around the resistance of a given PCP and strive to show how their services can add value to the care of patients. BHPs can demonstrate their skills in a variety of situations in the exam room, including handling tense situations between companions, distraught individuals, or someone trying to comprehend an overwhelming medical condition. Comparing outcome data between PCPs who embrace the model and those who do not can be enlightening to a PCP who does not yet appreciate the improvements that can be attained. Designing a system of care that provides PCPs with pocket protocols, a BHP at their side, and a consultant psychiatrist a phone call away can lead to an enhanced experience in caring for patients and an added sense of competence in treating behavioral health conditions. This coordinated system of "indirect" and "direct" consultation may take some time to perfect but once established can empower the PCP in recognizing and adequately treating a myriad of behavioral health conditions with the ongoing support of the BHP and consultant psychiatrist.

Case Example: Working With a Reluctant Primary Care Provider

Dr. Banner is a PCP in a rural federally qualified health center and has a large caseload of medically complicated patients. He is one of four providers in this clinic that decided to implement the Improving Mood—Promoting Access to Collaborative Treatment (IMPACT) model of collaborative care. At the first meeting, he stated up front that he did not have time to "add one more problem" to the list of issues he was trying to address at each visit and did not further investigate abnormal findings from the screening tools such as the PHQ-9 or seek out symptoms of emotional distress from his patients. He did not request the assistance of the BHP or introduce any patients via the "warm handoff" process. The BHP and psychiatrist continued to work with all the PCPs, discussing outcome data, providing education, and assisting in difficult situations. Dr. Banner listened to the stories presented in staff meetings about the successes of his colleagues and noted the interesting things that were beginning to happen. He noted how appreciative his colleagues were of the assistance they got from having the BHP on location and how they found the phone consultations with the psychiatrist to be very useful. One day he asked the BHP to help him in an emotionally charged session with a patient and was impressed with their handling of the situation and grateful he could move on to the next exam room. At the next staff meeting, he agreed to have the BHP meet some of his patients and agreed to scheduling follow-up appointments for patients with elevated PHQ-9 scores to separately address their depression. The psychiatrist and BHP looked across the table at each other and smiled in acknowledgment of their progress with this provider.

Consultant Psychiatrist

The role of the consultant psychiatrist will be more fully explored in Chapter 3 ("Role of the Consulting Psychiatrist") and has been mentioned in descriptions of the key tasks and relationships with other providers in this section. Psychiatrically trained nurse-practitioners and physician assistants may also participate on these teams in addition to psychiatrists but will likely not have the benefit of the in-depth education and experience that come with the knowledge psychiatrists receive over the course of medical school and psychiatric residency training. Some programs have utilized behavioral pharmacists in the absence of finding a consultant psychiatrist to provide some enhanced pharmacologic advice to PCPs and included them as an addition to the CC team.

Silent Partners

In addition to the traditional members of the CC team, a host of other important figures need to be recognized for their influence and contribution to the process. Receptionists, medical assistants, nurses, administrators, board members, and other staff are vital to the success of this process and provide needed additional support and participation in varying aspects of the model. Failure to appreciate their contribution can lead to disappointment, confusion, and poor outcomes. An example of this would be reception staff failing to make sure screening is taking place in the waiting room because of not wanting to "offend" patients, even though this is a vital prerequisite for measuring the subsequent steps in the treatment process. On the other hand, there may be "champions" of integration in this group who make the system work in remarkable ways, and they deserve recognition and nurturing. An example of this influence is a medical assistant who takes on the task of notifying the BHP in advance when there is a patient with a high screening score or when a more complicated appointment is anticipated based on his or her initial assessment. Sharing outcome data can help all staff understand the value of the model as well as identify ways they can enhance the treatment. This transparency around shared goals and outcomes is one of the ways to avoid conflict and can serve as a grounding force when confusion occurs. Everyone in the clinic plays a role on the CC team and engaging them in the excitement and rewards that come with knowing better care is being provided, as a result of the collective efforts of all of the staff, can be invaluable.

EVIDENCE-BASED BRIEF INTERVENTIONS OVERVIEW

This section will provide a review of some basics about the most commonly used evidence-based brief interventions in the primary care setting. These are short descriptions, and further information can be found in the resources suggested in each section. The brief interventions are matched to the patients' needs and preferences and often overlap to include elements of several techniques in a single session. While many of these brief interventions are recommended in sessions ranging from 4 to 12 weeks, the experience in primary care settings is that there may be only 1 or 2 sessions that actually occur, and the skilled BHP will maximize the potential of the limited time available to obtain the most benefit.

Motivational Interviewing

Motivational interviewing was first described by Miller and Rollnick (1991) and is a form of treatment that relies on a person's own beliefs around the change process. It follows three basic concepts: form a collaborative partnership, honor the patient's decisions regarding change, and elicit his or her reasons for change. Motivational interviewing differs from the usual care provided by many practitioners because it diverges from *dictating* to patients why they should change (e.g., "I advise you to stop smoking.") to *asking* them why they think they should change (e.g., "Why do you think you should stop smoking?"). Having patients decide why they should change a behavior and how they propose to do it (e.g., "How do you want to stop smoking?") has been shown in multiple trials to be effective across a variety of disorders (Rollnick et al. 2008) and is frequently utilized as an effective brief intervention by all members of the CC team.

Behavioral Activation

BA employs strategies to alter the environment in order to change how one feels (Lejuez et al. 2001). Life events can lead to feelings such as sadness and hopelessness, which, in turn, lead to maladaptive behaviors and worsening of symptoms (e.g., staying in bed, withdrawing from friends). This cycle serves to maintain the symptoms, and disrupting it by devising a list of pleasurable activities and having the patient agree to engage in them is the central feature of BA. The patient chooses one or more activities, tracks his or her progress, and reports to the therapist what he or she was able to accomplish and any barriers encountered. A simple exercise is to have the patient choose one activity he or she agrees to do in the coming week (e.g., walk to the park) and have the patient report at the next appointment (or by phone) if he or she accomplished this goal and how he or she felt. A new goal is then set for the following week. This technique is utilized frequently by BHPs because it can be done quickly in the primary care setting and has demonstrated effectiveness in the treatment of depression (Spates et al. 2006).

Problem-Solving Therapy

PST is similar to BA in the recognition that life problems lead to psychological distress, and it employs a strategy for systematic problem solving to find solutions (Mynors-Wallis et al. 2000). The provider and patient discuss problems the patient is currently experiencing, select one or more to address, and then follow a seven-step process to solve the problem(s). PST was the brief therapy chosen for the original IMPACT trial (Unützer et al. 2002) and a manual was developed for use during implementation and is available at http://impact-uw.org/training/problem_solving.html.

Distress Tolerance Skills

Distress tolerance skills are an important part of dialectical behavior therapy (Linehan 1993) and are useful in urgent situations where a solution may not be readily apparent or available. Four strategies are employed and can be easily taught in a brief intervention during an appointment in a primary care clinic, and one or more of these can be selected based on the presenting problem. They include utilizing techniques for *distraction* to take the focus off a situation, *self-soothing* through any of the five senses, *relaxation* techniques such as deep breathing, and assessing the *pros and cons* of reactions to stressful events to find a therapeutic alternative.

PUTTING IT ALL TOGETHER

The following vignette shows how the process works from screening and engagement to treatment and tracking for a patient receiving treatment from an evidence-based CC team.

Case Example: Putting the Steps Together

A.J. attends an appointment for her regular checkup for hypertension and hypothyroidism. While in the waiting room, she completes the PHQ-9, GAD-7, and the AUDIT. Her PHQ-9 score is 16 (high), her GAD-7 is 5 (normal), and her AUDIT is 0 (she does not drink). She is taken to the exam room, where her vitals are taken and recorded: a body mass index (BMI) of 27 (high), blood pressure 132/77, pulse 74, respirations 12, and temperature 98.6. Her PCP Dr. Smith enters the exam room and reviews her screening scores. He briefly asks about her increase in BMI from 26 to 27 since her last appointment and then asks a few follow-up questions because he also notices her PHQ-9 score is elevated. After a brief discussion, he discovers she has been struggling with low mood and lack of motivation for several years and that she was treated in the 1990s with amitriptyline for depression. She feels this may be contributing to her lack of exercise and subsequent recent increase in her weight. Dr. Smith steps out for a moment and knocks on the door of Sue Black, the clinic BHP, and has her join him for a discussion with A.J., introducing Sue as a member of the primary care team. Dr. Smith leaves the room to go see his next patient, and Sue questions A.J. in more detail about her symptoms, discovering a pattern consistent with the diagnosis of major depression. She evaluates her for any family history of mental disorders, symptoms of mania, trauma, substance use, and prior treatment. During the visit, she works with A.J., utilizing the brief intervention behavioral activation, and they develop an action plan where she will call two friends from her bike club in the next week. In addition, Sue provides her with educational material on sleep hygiene after discovering this has also been an issue. Sue excuses herself and finds Dr. Smith in an exam room down the hall. They speak briefly in the hallway about A.J. and decide an antidepressant in addition to several follow-up visits with Sue would be a good treatment approach. Dr. Smith and Sue go back into the exam room and discuss the plan with A.J., who consents to a trial of antidepressants, stating, "I've had problems with those medications in the past," revealing further history of several trials of selective serotonin reuptake inhibitors that resulted in weight gain. Dr. Smith is unsure what to do next and has Sue call the consultant psychiatrist, Dr. Green, who suggests a trial of bupropion SR 300 mg/day because it is less frequently associated with weight gain and may have the added benefit of appetite suppression. Dr. Green asks the BHP about head trauma, seizures, and any history of an eating disorder and warns Sue of potential problems with activation and insomnia and suggests having Dr. Smith call him if he has any questions. He also inquires if there is a recent thyroid-stimulating hormone level. The PCP and BHP discuss the treatment strategy together with A.J., who is agreeable with the plan. Sue adds A.J. to her registry, recording her baseline PHQ-9 score of 16. Dr. Smith decides to use the advice from the psychiatric consultant and writes a prescription for the bupropion. Sue calls A.J. the following week to see how she is feeling and if she made the calls to her friends. She also assesses her for sleep and tolerance of the bupropion. While on the phone, she has her complete the PHQ-9 and the score is now 12. This is recorded in the registry, and they make a plan to meet the following week for a brief office visit for another session of BA. She also confirms her follow-up appointment with Dr. Smith in 2 weeks to review her progress and the thyroid-stimulating hormone level that was obtained during her last visit. During her weekly caseload review with Dr. Green, they discuss A.J. and feel they have a good plan in place and will continue to monitor her progress with a PHQ target of < 5.

GETTING STARTED: DESIGNING A COLLABORATIVE CARE TEAM

It is important to remember the saying "If you've seen one integrated care team, you've seen one integrated care team" because local resources will often dictate how a program gets implemented in a given area. There are many excellent resources currently available from a variety of organizations to help design and implement an effective team. However, the most crucial step is the first one, which is to build interest and enthusiasm to encourage the adoption of the model. This is a vital aspect of success and typically involves garnering buy-in from at least two organizations because current models tend to pair the resources of an organization that provides primarily behavioral health services with a primary care group. One organization may approach the other with the intention of selling the idea, and every effort should be made to ensure there is broad agreement from senior management to the clinical and administrative staff. Experience has demonstrated that without this buy-in, and with the pressures of merging the disparate cultures of primary care and behavioral health, there can be a breakdown in the application of the core principles and resolve to carry the project forward (Bauer et al. 2011; Lardieri et al. 2014).

Once agreement is achieved, the next task is assessing the needs of the collaborating organizations and building the team around the resources that are available. There are numerous excellent resources available, including the Principles and Tasks Checklist from the Advancing Integrated Mental Health Solutions (AIMS) Center (http://uwaims.org/files/AIMS_Principles_Checklist_final.pdf). This Web site has numerous implementation resources, including measurement and tracking tools, online training modules for all members of the CC team, billing and finance information, and patient education materials. Another resource is the Substance Abuse and Mental Health Services Administration–Health Resources and Services Administration Center for Integrated Health Solutions (www. integration.samhsa.gov/), which has similar resources and a library of webinars on various topics related to integrated care that are available for viewing. The Center for Integrated Health Solutions is also the technical assistance center for the Primary and Behavioral Health Care Integration grantees (Chapter 8, "Providing Primary Care in Behavioral Health Settings") for organizations that are interested in improving the health status of patients with serious mental illnesses. The American Psychiatric Association has information and tools for psychiatrists working in integrated care settings (www.psych.org/practice/professional-interests/integrated-care). The Integrated Behavioral Health Project (www.ibhp.org/) developed Partners in Health: Mental Health, Primary Care and Substance Use Interagency Collaboration Tool Kit. Although tailored for the state of California, this 353-page document has an array of forms and measurement tools in addition to links to helpful resources that can be used nationwide. There are numerous organizations that provide individual consultation services to organizations wishing to build an integrated care program.

TEAM DYNAMICS AT THE INTERFACE OF PRIMARY CARE AND BEHAVIORAL HEALTH

The essence of integrated care is a well-functioning team. Building an effective CC team requires more than simply putting multidisciplinary providers together in a clinic and assigning them tasks along the stepped-care ladder. Integrated and collaborative care requires the intersection of two previously "siloed" treatment systems and has numerous limitations to overcome. On the basis of a long history of conceptually different cultures (i.e., biomedical versus biopsychosocial) and a distinct separation of provider training, communication, delivery of services, and funding systems, deep-rooted boundaries exist between physical and behavioral health treatment providers and systems. The team of providers must then overcome these cultural boundaries, shift their practice, and develop an entirely new treatment approach. These are genuine paradigm shifts for both organizations and individuals and should not be underestimated.

As team-based care gains attention across health care settings, numerous entities have attempted to delineate components of effective health care teams. The Institute of Medicine's (IOM's) core principles and values of effective team-based health care outline consistent elements across teams, including the following: patient and family involvement, with each being viewed as team members; the use of more than one clinician or discipline; team-based identification of preferred treatment goals; close coordination across settings; and clear communication with structured feedback channels. The authors outline a set of core principles of effective team-based care (see Table 2–7) and discuss the five personal values most frequently exhibited by providers on highly functioning teams, which include honesty, humility, creativity, discipline, and curiosity (Mitchell et al. 2012).

More recently, the IOM released a document describing the pressures and necessities within health care to move toward team-based care. They in-

---

TABLE 2–7.   Principles of team-based health care

1. **Shared goals:** The team—including the patient and, where appropriate, family members or other support persons—works to establish shared goals that reflect patient and family priorities and that can be clearly articulated, understood, and supported by all team members.

2. **Clear roles:** There are clear expectations for each team member's functions, responsibilities, and accountabilities, which optimize the team's efficiency and often make it possible for the team to take advantage of division of labor, thereby accomplishing more than the sum of its parts.

3. **Mutual trust:** Team members earn each other's trust, creating strong norms of reciprocity and greater opportunities for shared achievement.

4. **Effective communication:** The team prioritizes and continuously refines its communication skills. It has consistent channels for candid and complete communication, which are accessed and used by all team members across all settings.

5. **Measurable processes and outcomes:** The team agrees on and implements reliable and timely feedback on successes and failures in both the functioning of the team and achievement of the team's goals. These are used to track and improve performance immediately and over time.

Source.   Reprinted from Mitchell P, Wynia M, Golden R, et al.: "Core Principles & Values of Effective Team-Based Health Care." Discussion Paper. Washington, DC, Institute of Medicine, 2012, p. 6. Copyright 2012.

---

troduce a concept of transdisciplinary professionalism that highlights the importance of interprofessional teamwork, measurable outcomes, and accountability for population health. The authors defined *transdisciplinary professionalism* as "an approach to creating and carrying out a shared social contract that ensures multiple health disciplines, working in concert, are worthy of the trust of patients and the public *in order to improve the health of patients and their communities*" (National Research Council 2013, p. 1).

A pilot study looking at essential elements of teams integrating primary care and behavioral health found many of the same themes, demonstrating there is broad consistency about what makes an effective CC team (Lardieri et al. 2014). The four Essential Elements of Integrated Primary and Behavioral Health Care teams describe some attributes that are unique to integrated care in addition to the IOM principles mentioned above. This study demonstrated that it is vital to have strong *leadership* and *organizational commitment* to the philosophy of integrated care in order for teams to thrive and for the model to be fully developed. A second consistent theme is the need for considerable time and energy focused on formal and informal *team development,* with joint primary care and behavioral health staff participation, to break down some of the culture barriers. Team development focuses on issues such as creating a team vision, team values, fostering relationships among team members, hiring the "right providers," and clarifying roles and responsibilities of team members. As the IOM found, a third key element is effective communication, which is vital to collaborative care teams. Communication takes various forms, including clinical case review, day-to-day operational concerns and patient care, and process communication regarding how well the team is meeting shared treatment goals. In addition, CC teams need to continually assess the *team process* and address areas of conflict or reduced team functionality due in part to misunderstandings that may arise as a result of their cultural differences. The fourth and final principle is that successful CC teams use patient *outcomes* to assess the treatment provided and make needed changes to obtain previously defined and shared outcomes. It is often this last element that allows the merging cultures of primary care and behavioral health to move past conflicts and confusion when the team uses predetermined patient outcomes as the yardstick for determining success regardless of discipline or intervention.

There are unique aspects of CC team development that require focused attention by both organizational leaders and individual providers. For example, cross-training of providers becomes far more important in CC as medical providers understand behavioral health and BHPs learn vital health indicators. One way to make this cultural shift real is to demonstrate the behaviors required for collaboration. As described in the section "Behavioral Health Providers," developing a shadowing tool for each team member and his or her discipline can facilitate more effective training and operation of the model. This is a practical way to help providers shift paradigms in clinical practice. In addition, because the medical and behavioral health organizations have a long history of siloed systems of funding, billing structures, and cadence of work flow, there is a need for specific system and operational support of integrated care teams. These operational supports provide the essential "back end" support that allows for billing and documentation in this innovative model of care (Lardieri et al. 2014).

CONCLUSION

Effective collaborative care teams adhere to a set of core principles and tasks that guide their successful implementation. Careful attention to the selection of team members who have the skills and attitude necessary to perform these functions is crucial to realizing the outcomes that are possible as demonstrated by the evidence base for these models. The success of the program also hinges on astute leadership that understands the dynamics of teams and the inherent friction that occurs when cultures unite to provide whole-person care.

REFERENCES

Bauer A, Azzone E, Goldman H, et al: Implementation of collaborative depression management at community-based primary care clinics: an evaluation. Psychiatr Serv 62(9):1047–1053, 2011

Folstein MF, Folstein SE, McHugh PR: "Mini-mental state": a practical method for grading the cognitive states of patients for the clinician. J Psychiatr Res 12(3):189–198, 1975

Fortney JC, Pyne JM, Mouden SB, et al: Practice-based versus telemedicine-based collaborative care for depression in rural federally qualified health centers: a pragmatic randomized comparative effectiveness trial. Am J Psychiatry 170:414–425, 2013

Gavin DR, Ross HE, Skinner HA: Diagnostic validity of the Drug Abuse Screening Test in the assessment of DSM-III drug disorders. Br J Addict 84:301–307, 1989

Hirschfeld RM, Williams JB, Spitzer RL, et al: Development and validation of a screening instrument for bipolar spectrum disorder: the Mood Disorders Questionnaire. Am J Psychiatry 157:1873–1875, 2000

Katon WJ, Lin EH, Von Korff M, et al: Collaborative care for patients with depression and chronic illnesses. N Engl J Med 363(27):2611–2620, 2010

Kroenig K, Spitzer RL: The PHQ-9: validity of a brief depression severity measure. J Intern Med 16(9):606–613, 2001

Lardieri M, Lasky G, Raney L: Essential elements of integrated primary and behavioral health teams. Washington, DC, SAMHSA-HRSA Center for Integrated Health Solutions, 2014. Available at: http://www.integration.samhsa.gov/workforce/team-members/Essential_Elements_of_an_Integrated_Team.pdf. Accessed March 6, 2014.

Lejuez CW, Hopko DR, Hopko SD: A brief behavioral activation treatment for depression. Behav Modif 25(2):255–286, 2001

Levine S, Unützer J, Yip JY, et al: Physicians' satisfaction with a collaborative disease management program for late-life depression in primary care. Gen Hosp Psychiatry 27:383– 391, 2005

Linehan M: Skills Training Manual for Treating Borderline Personality Disorder. New York, Guilford, 1993

Miller WR, Rollnick S: Motivational Interviewing: Preparing People for Change. New York, Guilford, 1991

Mitchell P, Wynia M, Golden R, et al: Core Principles & Values of Effective Team-Based Health Care. Discussion Paper. Washington, DC, Institute of Medicine, 2012. Available at: https://www.nationalahec.org/pdfs/VSRT-Team-Based-Care-Principles-values.pdf. Accessed December 12, 2013.

Mynors-Wallis LM, Day GD, Baker F: Randomised controlled trial of problem solving treatment, antidepressant medication, and combined treatment for depression in primary care. BMJ 320(7226):26–30, 2000

National Research Council: Establishing Transdisciplinary Professionalism for Improving Health Outcomes: Workshop Summary. Washington, DC, National Academies Press, 2013. Available at: http://www.nap.edu/catalog.php?record_id=18398. Accessed December 12, 2013.

Olfson M, Fireman B, Weissman M, et al: Mental disorders and disability among patients in a primary care group practice. Am J Psychiatry 155:1734–1740, 1997

Prins A, Ouimette P, Kimerling R, et al: The primary care PTSD screen (PC-PTSD): development and operating characteristics. Primary Care Psychiatry 9(1):9–14, 2003

Rollnick S, Miller WR, Butler CC: Motivational Interviewing in Health Care: Helping Patients Change Behavior. New York, Guilford, 2008

Saunders JB, Aasland OG, Babor TF, et al: Development of the Alcohol Use Disorders Identification Test (AUDIT): WHO Collaborative Project on Early Detection of Persons with Harmful Alcohol Consumption—II. Addiction 88(6):791–804, 1993

Spates CR, Pagoto S, Kalata A: A qualitative and quantitative review of behavioral activation treatment of major depressive disorder. Behav Anal Today 7(4):508–518, 2006

Spitzer RL, Kroenke K, Williams JB: A brief measure for assessing generalized anxiety disorder: the GAD-7. Arch Intern Med 166(10):1092–1097, 2006

Unützer J, Katon W, Callahan CM, et al: Collaborative-care management of late-life depression in the primary care setting. JAMA 288(22):2836–2845, 2002

Von Korff M, Tiemens B: Individualized stepped care of chronic illnesses. West J Med 172(2):133–137, 2000

CHAPTER 3

Role of the Consulting Psychiatrist

Lori Raney, M.D.

> Leadership is about staking your ground ahead of where opinion is and convincing people, not simply following the popular opinion of the moment.
>
> Doris Kearns Goodwin

In Chapter 2 ("The Collaborative Care Team in Action"), the key members of the collaborative care (CC) team and the specific tasks for the primary care provider (PCP) and behavioral health provider (BHP) were identified. This chapter will explore the roles of the psychiatric consultant, which consist of a diverse range of activities, including providing informal consultation, direct evaluation of patients, education, population-based care, and leadership. Psychiatrists are uniquely suited to lead teams in the primary care setting and ensure team cohesiveness, spanning the historically separate cultures of primary care and behavioral health that has proven to be one of the greatest challenges to effective implementation. Effective psychiatric consultation will be an asset to primary care organizations pursuing certification as patient-centered medical homes (PCMHs), with their emphasis on managing multiple chronic conditions, including behavioral health disorders.

ROLES FOR THE CONSULTANT PSYCHIATRIST

Informal "Curbside" Consultation

Readily accessible "curbside" or informal psychiatric consultation is a cornerstone of effective collaboration. It allows patients to be treated at the time of their primary care appointment rather than postponing to a later stage and further delaying treatment. Prior to contacting the consultant psychiatrist, the BHP and PCP will have gathered useful information, including medical history, results of behavioral health screenings, laboratory results, and other clinical data, and the BHP will have completed a brief assessment of the patient. As the patient moves through the levels of the stepped-care ladder (described in Chapter 2), a point will be reached where specialist input is needed to deliver immediate and effective care, and communication with the consulting psychiatrist is then initiated.

The most common reasons for consultation are requests for psychopharmacologic recommendations or diagnostic clarification. Frequently, consultation requires sorting through the various ways psychiatric symptoms present in primary care and the medical conditions that may mimic them. Common diagnostic categories for these consultations include depression, anxiety, bipolar disorder, personality disorders, substance use, and somatization disorders. Although there is not a robust evidence base for CC models for disorders other than depression and anxiety, patients present with a variety of conditions, and this should not limit the psychiatrist's involvement in assisting the team. The first study looking at the treatment of bipolar disorder in primary care settings using the CC model demonstrated that more intensive care is needed for this population. Only one third experienced clinically meaningful improvement, demonstrated by changes in the Patient Health Questionnaire depression rating scale (PHQ-9) and the seven-item Generalized Anxiety Disorder Scale (GAD-7); more specialty behavioral health care, either through on-site services or by referral, will most likely be necessary to improve outcomes (Cerimele et al., 2014). Given that primary care clinics are often staffed by family practice providers, requests for consultation across the life span, from pediatrics to geriatrics, are common, and the psychiatrist may need to broaden his or her skill set to be able to provide this consultation, with backup from a child psychiatrist or other specialty-trained colleagues as needed. Requests for consultation for substance use, chronic pain, and geriatric disorders are also common. Similar to family practice physicians, consultant psychiatrists should endeavor to be "generalists" as much as possible, with additional training in areas where there is less comfort with their skill set (see Chapter 4, "Child and Adolescent Psychiatry in Integrated Settings," section "Adult Psychiatrists Consulting in Pediatric Primary Care"). Psychiatric providers are encouraged to closely follow the literature as this field continues to evolve and new approaches to treating behavioral health conditions in primary care settings are published and become evidence-based practices.

Experience to date has been that these consultations can be completed in a manageable period of time, averaging around 5 minutes apiece (J. Kern, M.D., personal communication, October 2013). The number and complexity of consultation requests depend on the size of the clinic and level of behavioral health severity in the population. For instance, federally qualified health centers tend to serve indigent populations who have higher rates of mental illness, and factoring in more time for consultations is usually necessary, while in clinics with more privately insured patients, the demand for consultation may be less. These consultations may be undertaken in a variety of ways, including by mobile phone, texting, or e-mail communication between the BHP, the PCP, and the psychiatric consultant depending on their preferences. Consultant psychiatrists should be expected to return calls in a timely manner, usually within 1–2 hours if they are not answered immediately, and strive to provide coverage for absences to provide consistency to the primary care team. Last, these consultations may be works in progress, and the consultant psychiatrist will need to achieve some level of comfort with making recommendations on the basis of the available information, which may initially be incomplete and added to over time.

Working with PCPs first and foremost requires they know you "have their backs" as they go about the process of diagnosing and treating behavioral health conditions that they are uncomfortable with and may feel are outside their area of expertise. Nudging them along, encouraging them to go beyond first- and second-line treatments, while having the patients remain in the primary care setting, all have a better chance of succeeding if PCPs trust you are readily accessible. This type of support from psychiatry will be new (and unexpected) to most PCPs and will require some emphasizing for a successful partnership.

The liability incurred while doing informal consultations is often a concern for psychiatrists beginning work in collaborative settings; this is more fully explored in Chapter 5 ("Risk Management and Liability Issues in Integrated Care"). Current literature and case law suggest the risk is minimal (Olick and Bergus 2003) and should not deter psychiatrists from participating. While it is less common for the consulting psychiatrist to write a note detailing an informal consultation, if this should occur it is recommended a disclaimer statement be added explaining that the patient was not directly evaluated. As explained in Chapter 5, it is also advisable that the care of the patient remain under the direction of the PCP, who may or may not choose to use the advice offered in an informal consultation. He or she can "take it or leave it" and should also remain in charge of ordering medications and additional testing or services.

Formal Consultation or Direct Patient Evaluation

A limited consultation role for the psychiatrist is the direct evaluation of patients who have moved through the stepped-care system and are not improving. In the original Improving Mood—Promoting Access to Collaborative Treatment (IMPACT) trial, approximately 95% of patients were treated utilizing the care given by the PCP and BHP with informal consultation from the psychiatrist, and the remaining 5%–7% of patients who had more difficult presentations and were not responding to treatment received direct evaluation (Unützer et al. 2002). These evaluations can occur on-site in the primary care setting or from a distance by televideo and often consist of one or two appointments with the patient to provide recommendations to the team. They also can permit an opportunity for both the BHP and the PCP to participate in the interview if time and interest allow, further enhancing their knowledge of a psychiatrist's approach to diagnostic interviewing and treatment planning. It is important for the BHP to be the gatekeeper for the psychiatrist's direct evaluation time to ensure patients have moved through the stepped-care system first and have not simply been referred for specialist consultation by a busy or reluctant PCP who does not want to manage a particular behavioral health condition. If colocation is allowed to occur, the psychiatric provider will quickly build a caseload of patients referred from the PCP, which will restrict access and result in extended waits for appointments and frustrated PCPs. With this method in place, psychiatric resources can be extended to a larger population of patients and prevent colocation, which would just perpetuate the current limitations of access to psychiatric expertise. This is crucial to the model and must be strictly adhered to.

It is important for the psychiatrist to document any direct assessments (either face-to-face or by televideo) in the patient's primary care medical record, using standard evaluation and management coding and utilizing a format that collects and records facts without overly describing sensitive information resembling that found in a typical psychiatric evaluation. This protects a patient's privacy around delicate matters while gathering crucial details to arrive at a diagnosis and treatment plan (e.g., "B.F. has a history of trauma as a child" vs. "B.F. was sexually abused by her father and uncle from the ages of 8 to 11"). This also limits the length of the written evaluation to a briefer version that is more likely to be read by a busy PCP. Some psychiatrists utilize an APSO approach to the typical SOAP note (subjective, objective, assessment, plan), placing the diagnosis (assessment) followed by treatment recommendations (plan) at the top of the progress note, with the remainder of the information (subjective and objective findings) at the end. A PCP may or may not read the latter part of the evaluation but can quickly incorporate treatment recommendations in this format. It is important to include specifics on side effects, recommendations for alternatives, next steps, and titration information since this is usually a one-time evaluation by the psychiatric consultant, with the PCP continuing the patient care. Every consultation is also an opportunity for education, so additional information that may be useful in the PCP's or BHP's treatment of other patients with similar conditions is an added benefit.

Psychiatrists are often concerned about the Health Insurance Portability and Accountability Act (HIPAA) and 42 C.F.R. (Code of Federal Regulations implementing federal drug and alcohol information confidentiality law 42 U.S.C. 290dd-2) as they pertain to the sharing of mental health and substance use information in the primary care setting. CC teams are often formed through agreement between two organizations such as a community mental health center and primary care clinic (often a federally qualified health center) partnership. Although some states may have more stringent privacy laws, HIPAA allows the sharing of information obtained by the psychiatrist and BHP with the primary care clinic staff because the two agencies are considered "business associates" and are sharing information to "coordinate care." In an arrangement where the psychiatrist is directly hired by the primary care clinic, he or she is a member of the same staff, and HIPAA is not an issue, but care in writing the notes, as mentioned above, is suggested. In the 42 C.F.R. regulations, what is specifically prohibited without a signed release from the patient is the release of information *from* a drug and alcohol treatment or prevention program or speciality provider. It is not necessary for a substance abuse counselor working with the CC team to shield his or her notes from the rest of the team. If there is a request for information from an outside organization, then the substance use counseling notes only would require a written release from the patient. This will be more fully covered in Chapter 5 on liability and is important to understand because these two regulations are frequently misinterpreted and hinder successful integration. Consultant psychiatrists should acquaint themselves with the privacy regulations of their state and of the organizations in which they provide consultation, because they may be more stringent than federal governmental regulations for HIPAA.

Population-Based Care

Population-based care is one of the CC core principles and represents a significant divergence from the traditional way psychiatrists have approached patient care. Moving from an individual and autonomous method of providing one-on-one care for individual patients requesting treatment to a system where responsibility for the detection and treatment of conditions in a defined population of patients is the approach may take some getting used to by traditionally trained psychiatrists. This involves first screening the select population (this could be for behavioral health conditions in settings such as primary care or screening for general medical conditions in groups with serious mental illnesses), followed by tracking and reviewing aggregate data for care gaps and progress toward goals. Predetermined data points, such as PHQ-9 scores, are collected in a tracking instrument called a registry (covered in Chapter 2). This format allows for easy review (and sorting of data if electronic) to determine who is not improving, who has missed appointments, and where follow-up is needed. On the basis of these data, treatment changes are recommended to intensify management and improve the chances of an effective response. High utilizers and high-cost patients can be tracked, which is an important component of being accountable for the care provided. These data can also be used to assess the overall performance of the program for both clinical and administrative purposes, such as the percentage of patients who experienced a 50% or more drop in PHQ-9 scores or a goal of 65% or more of patients who were not showing improvement receiving a psychiatric consultation. Individual provider's performance can also be measured and compared, and this review process is vital to tracking quality measures used in pay-for-performance programs. The consulting psychiatrist is instrumental in this process because he or she participates in the data review and can discover any gaps in care and can define opportunities to improve outcomes by adjusting treatment. This disciplined approach by the team can lead to better outcomes and accountability for the care provided.

Regular review of the registry by the BHP and psychiatrist occurs at a weekly, biweekly, or monthly frequency depending on the size of the caseload and severity of the problems. This may occur in person, over the phone, or by televideo depending on distance and equipment available. It could also begin with an in-person review if the psychiatrist does not yet know the BHP, or their skill level, and progress to using other forms of communication as the relationship and mutual trust develop. The BHP should come prepared for these meetings with copies of the registry available or on-screen for joint review, with a column reserved to record the psychiatrist's recommendations and another with current medications to assist in making any suggested medication changes. With this information, the BHP and psychiatric provider can move efficiently through the registry, reviewing from 10 to 20 patients over the course of an hour, discussing those who are not improving and treatment changes needed or deciding who might need a direct evaluation by the psychiatrist (Table 3–1).

This registry review component, in addition to the curbside and direct evaluations, allows a remarkable amount of psychiatric expertise to be de-

TABLE 3–1. Example of registry review with behavioral health provider and recommendations recorded

Reason for consultation	Diagnoses	Recommendations
Side effects from lithium	Bipolar I	Switch to valproic acid
Increased depression	MDD	Increase dose, consider switch to bupropion
Side effects from stimulant	ADHD	Try another stimulant per protocol
Suicidal, acute distress	Personality disorder	Safety plan and therapy
Depression increased	Bipolar I	Check lithium level, add lamotrigine if in range
High doses of medications, confused	MDD	Reduce lorazepam, stop hydroxyzine, get collateral information
Anxious, wants alprazolam	GAD	No alprazolam, increase sertraline, coping skills

Note. ADHD=attention-deficit/hyperactivity disorder; GAD=generalized anxiety disorder; MDD=major depressive disorder.

livered to a clinic population. The scalability of this concept is not yet clear, but one estimate of psychiatric time needed ranges from approximately 1 to 2 hours a week for a clinic population of 2,000 patients (with a subset of patients with moderate levels of mental illness). The number of hours of consultant time increases in safety net populations, where there is a higher incidence of behavioral health disorders and more frequent contact will be necessary. Given the current shortage of psychiatrists, this model provides an excellent way to employ limited psychiatric resources for a larger population of patients utilizing an evidence-based approach.

Education

Every consultation request presents an opportunity for teaching. PCPs are typically interested in assistance with medication recommendations, and one way to help them is to include the rationale for a particular treatment as it is being recommended. A brief phone call may include a recommendation for a specific antidepressant and an explanation of why that particular one was chosen. Regular involvement with administrative and other clinical staff is also invaluable and when used to shore up administrative support for the collaborative model can be one of the most important interventions of the consultant psychiatrist. The team may also want to consider joint attendance at trainings or conferences or other settings that allow shared learning on a topic of interest in the CC arena.

Case Example: Informal Consultation With an Educational Component

You receive a call from Dr. Smith who has a patient with depression and chronic pain who is currently prescribed bupropion 300 mg/day and has a PHQ-9 score of 16 after 7 weeks on medication (his baseline score was 24). He experienced some jitteriness on 450 mg, and the dose was reduced to 300 mg. He has been on sertraline and fluoxetine in the past without response, and Dr. Smith asks you what she should do next. You suggest venlafaxine starting at 75 mg and titrating up to 150 mg over the course of the next week and further 75-mg increases every 4–6 weeks until his PHQ-9 score falls below 5. You go on to explain to Dr. Smith that you chose venlafaxine for its dual action on both the serotonin and norepinephrine systems, which can be helpful with depression and chronic pain. You add that this combination would affect the norepinephrine, dopamine, and serotonin systems in the brain, and this combination may result in better efficacy for this patient. You also add that concurrent use of narcotics for chronic pain will inhibit the effectiveness because of their central nervous system depressant effects. You suggest she try this combination and call you if she has any further questions.

In addition to providing this information during the curbside consultation, the consultant psychiatrist may provide the PCP with algorithms for the treatment of common mental illnesses, including depression and anxiety. Over time, as the PCP becomes proficient in the treatment of these disorders, he or she may request guidance for other conditions such as bipolar or attention-deficit disorder. Creating or utilizing existing algorithms can give you a reference point in your discussions with the PCP and can move him or her toward competence in this area. Other opportunities to teach PCPs include "stump the chump" sessions where they ask about specific patients, presentations on topics of their choice (or areas of targeted educational needs you have discovered through your data review), and providing journal articles or Web site links and information on upcoming conferences. Covisits with patients provide another opportunity for education and are encouraged whenever possible. Over time, as the team becomes more confident with first- and second-line treatments, consultation requests are for more challenging scenarios.

Education for the BHPs tends to include more time spent on diagnostic clarification and treatment recommendations because they are the "boots on the ground" and the conveyors of information between the on-site team and the psychiatrist. Similar to the interactions with the PCP, many consultations present an opportunity for teaching, and every effort should be made to include this whenever possible. This teaching may include information on specific medical conditions and the differential diagnosis of the presenting symptoms of psychological distress in primary care settings. Differing levels of education and experience are also seen among BHPs, and the psychiatrist may find himself or herself instructing them in areas such as the basics of brief interventions and how to do concise presentations. Determining their skill level is an important task because the confidence of the PCPs in integrated settings often rests on their comfort level with the abilities of the BHP. Early efforts to discover any knowledge deficits and resolve them quickly through additional teaching are imperative. It is essential for the psychiatrist to convey confidence in the BHP in the presence of the PCP, and efforts should be made not to overcorrect or to unnecessarily demonstrate superiority in joint interactions. As one astute PCP said, "If you make yourself look smarter than the BHP, then you've made a mistake." It is also important for the BHP to fully understand how the CC model operates so he or she adheres to it when pressured to regress to a more colocated model. The BHP must have the knowledge and tenacity to withstand this and be a voice for fidelity to the model in order to leverage the available psychiatric expertise across the broader population. The consultant psychiatrist can guide him or her in this endeavor through training and coaching around the core principles (discussed in Chapter 1, "Evidence Base and Core Principles") and the core components of these evidence-based models. Last, it is important to understand that everyone contributes to the learning process. The consultant psychiatrist is constantly presented with opportunities to learn as well as teach. This is one of the many rewards of the psychiatric provider role.

Case Example: Collaborative Care Team Meeting

Dr. Scott is the consultant psychiatrist on a CC team at a federally qualified health center. She makes a monthly visit to this clinic, spending the first hour during breakfast in a staff meeting that includes the clinic administrator, PCPs, and the BHP. Today a new BHP and a new PCP are joining the existing team. Dr. Scott spends the first 30 minutes going over a diagram of the CC model, describing the core principles, the stepped-care approach, and the key functions of each team member and how she will interact with the team. She makes every effort to distinguish how this differs from a colocated model and discusses the importance of the registry to track patients and identify those in need of intensification of treatment to reach targeted end points. She gives the PCPs her mobile phone number and assures them she is there to assist in real time with their questions. She informs the team she will be conducting regular reviews with the BHP to discuss patients who are not improving and provide recommendations that the BHP will relay to the providers. The next 15 minutes is spent answering questions the PCPs may have about patients they have recently encountered, and the last 15 minutes is spent on the topic of pain management, which was determined to be an area for targeted educational intervention during a quarterly registry review. She finishes the meeting on time so the PCPs are not late for their first appointment. The next 30 minutes is spent with the BHP reviewing the registry, with the BHP presenting 15 patients who are new or not reaching treatment targets. The BHP and Dr. Scott come up with a plan for 14 of the patients, and Dr. Scott decides to see one patient on the next visit to the clinic. Dr. Scott spends the next 30 minutes of her 2-hour clinic visit directly evaluating a patient who has not been responding to treatment and documents her note in the electronic medical record for the PCP to read and follow the recommendations if desired.

Leadership

The two traditionally separate cultures of primary care and behavioral health come into contact with each other in new ways in CC programs. The skillful consultant psychiatrist will anticipate and be prepared to manage the inevitable tension that will arise. Once the model and benefits of integrating behavioral health into a primary care clinic have been explained, there is usually an initial eagerness to try the CC model. However, problems will occur when the PCP, BHP, and psychiatric provider have to actually change the way they have been historically practicing patient care and when staff, including the "silent partners" mentioned in Chapter 2, need to alter their work flows and belief systems to accommodate the model. As one observer noted, "Everyone wants to do integrated care until they have to change the way they practice." Differences in language, clinic pace, approaches to patient care, and other characteristics (see Table 2–1 in Chapter 2) will need close attention, and a willingness to openly discuss how to manage differing opinions and approaches to patient care is essential. It is important for the team to maintain fidelity to the model in order for it to work, because the pull to regress to colocation is stronger than often realized in the start-up phase. Colocation differs from most traditional psychiatric practices mainly by the close proximity to primary care (on-site). Whereas other resources may be shared (scheduling, electronic health records, etc.), problems with high no-show rates, full caseloads, and long waits for psychiatric appointments usually occur in colocated arrangements as time goes by, resulting in a replication of the current system of referring to psychiatrists for care.

There is potential for conflict at the administrative level if there is an absence of a shared mission through the ranks of management, clerical, nursing, billing, and other key staff. For example, problems can occur if a receptionist does not reliably make sure all patients are handed screening instruments, so the flow of referrals to the BHP is limited, and patients with mental distress are missed. Clinic administrators may not understand the need for team processing and cross-training to occur and may feel team meetings are not valuable enough to compensate for lost PCP productivity and therefore may not make time for the PCPs to attend.

Working with BHPs and PCPs requires some vigilance, especially early in the relationship when they are working to establish trust in each other. Conflicts sometimes arise around differing ideas about treatment that are inherent in the cultural differences they each bring to the work, and it is an important task for the psychiatrist to be watchful and skillfully intervene when necessary. Burnout, inappropriate requests of the BHP (for instance, to do clerical or case management–type work), and BHPs who are doing extended appointments with patients and not wanting to be interrupted are all issues that can arise and need to be addressed promptly so that the CC model can work effectively. Finding time for the team to meet together is crucial to these developing relationships and often difficult with the productivity demands in busy primary care clinics. The psychiatric consultant can play a vital role in the successful development of these teams if he or she recognizes the conflicts and barriers and strives to find solutions.

In the clinical space, if the PCP and BHP do not trust each other, conflict can occur as mentioned above, or a PCP can be so resistant to the model that nursing and other staff join forces and impede the process. It is important for there to be a leveling of the traditional hierarchy seen in the medical field to allow equal opportunity for all members of the CC team to provide input. In addition, placing a psychiatric provider on the team who is reluctant to provide curbside consultations because of liability concerns, or who does not return phone calls in a timely manner, can undermine the system considerably because the ability to make immediate adjustments in care will be lost in addition to PCP trust in the process.

The consultant psychiatrist will need to be prepared for and expect these difficulties and employ approaches to find solutions. One strategy is to find and nurture the champions of integration in the clinic, who could range from a receptionist to a medical assistant or the PCP. These cheerleaders can be powerful in spreading enthusiasm to the team and encouraging other staff to join the effort. Buy-in must flow from the board and executive leadership of the organization to the trenches where the actual collaboration is carried out. The importance of this component cannot be overstated (see Chapter 2).

An interesting study (Bauer et al. 2011) demonstrated how outcomes may be affected by these intangible properties. Clinics that received identical training and postimplementation consultation and had similar patient characteristics showed strikingly different clinical outcomes (Figure 3–1). The authors speculated that better clinical outcomes were seen in clinics in which the staff embraced the CC model and enacted the steps necessary for it to be successful. For example, one clinic had an administration that did not support the model, while another had a preexisting behavioral health team that appeared reluctant to change the way they were willing to provide care. Another team had a group that championed the model and strove to reach established goals despite obstacles in the organization.

It is imperative that there is an oversight mechanism to keep the team faithful to the principles and specific tasks of the CC model. This presents an

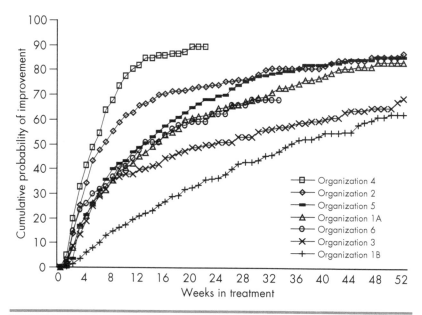

FIGURE 3–1.   Varying results at sites implementing a collaborative care model.
Estimated time elapsed between initial assessment and improvement of depression during the
first year of treatment at six organizations. Estimates were truncated when 10 or fewer patients
remained in treatment at each site.
Source.   Reprinted from Bauer AM, Azzone V, Goldman HH, et al.: "Implementation of Collaborative Management at Community-Based Primary Care Clinics: An Evaluation." *Psychiatric Services* 62(9):1047–1053, 2011. Used with permission. Copyright © 2011 American
Psychiatric Association.

opportunity for psychiatric leadership to help maintain fidelity to the model
while navigating the team dynamics that will most likely occur once the
model is up and running. The unique training psychiatrists have in both the
behavioral health and general medical fields provides them with the knowledge to speak the language of those on both sides of the boundary and to
work to resolve disagreements and misunderstandings. Education and experience with group dynamics will be valuable, and it is perhaps best to predict
in advance that difficulties will naturally emerge when two different cultures
come in contact with each other and to see this as an expected part of the
process to avoid becoming discouraged. It is potentially the leadership of the
astute psychiatrist that will help the team work through problems and develop the shared trust necessary so the most robust outcomes can be
achieved and satisfaction with the model ensues. Individuals working in effective CC teams often find this work very professionally rewarding and may
desire to work exclusively in these settings. The psychiatric consultant can
contribute by removing barriers and overcoming obstacles to help these

teams function successfully and can experience the satisfaction of knowing his or her leadership contributed to the team's success.

Psychiatric Consultant Experiences

Consulting in primary care has been a wonderful time off the hamster wheel of 15-minute med checks.

...a chance to use the full scope of my medical training, the ability to intervene on behalf of more patients than I can personally see, and helping to train other team members.

...to be involved in shaping the provision of mental health care for a large population of patients in primary care.

...to teach.

Leadership Approaches

There are numerous approaches to leadership, but several may be more relevant to the integration and cross-boundary work necessary for successful CC teams. Brief descriptions of two of the most central approaches are described here, with the reader encouraged to seek further information if desired.

Boundary-spanning leadership provides an interesting approach to leadership for psychiatrists who find themselves straddling the stances of the medical and behavioral health worlds and who witness what transpires when these two cultures bump up against one another. There are two ways to define a boundary: one as a type of border or limitation and the other as a frontier where new possibilities may exist. Boundary-spanning leadership is defined as "the ability to create direction, alignment, and commitment across boundaries in service of a higher vision or goal"; it is leadership that proposes that this "frontier" is a place of "limitless possibilities and inspiring results groups can achieve together, above and beyond what they can achieve alone" (Ernst and Chrobot-Mason 2011, p. 5). The process involves three stages that utilize specific tools. The first is managing boundaries, utilizing the tools buffering and reflecting to create safety and respect between groups (e.g., building safety and experimentation by allowing a team time to practice a huddle or new work flow without the immediate pressure of a full schedule). The second is forging common ground, utilizing the tools connecting and mobilizing to build trust and reframe boundaries (e.g., building trust by helping a provider group develop shared goals and focusing on the common goals and skills across traditional boundaries and developing trust by finding the common passion among providers to help a specific population). The last step is discovering new frontiers by using the tools weaving and transforming, which integrate groups into a new entity and enable reinvention of a new culture (e.g., focusing on the innovation and genuine growth in medical practice that can occur as a result of combining discipline strengths and differences into a unified group). While this is not a complete description of the process, the principles could be very useful concepts for leaders working to create successful CC teams (Ernst and Chrobot-Mason 2011).

Shared leadership is another important concept for team-based work that fits well with integrating care. It occurs "when all members of a team are fully engaged in leadership of the team and are not hesitant to influence and guide their fellow team members in an effort to maximize the potential of the team" (Pearce 2004, p. 48). While acknowledging there is also a need for vertical leadership (top-down process, one person "in charge"), there are three scenarios where shared leadership can be particularly successful. These include 1) teams that have a high interdependence on each other (such as CC teams); 2) tasks that require a lot of creativity where input from multiple individuals is more productive; and 3) projects that are very complex, where no one individual is likely to have all the answers for every component of an assignment. A leader who embraces this model will work to design an effective team, articulate the vision, clarify the purpose of the group, select members, and help manage boundaries while allowing the group members the freedom to exercise their individual expertise (Pearce 2004). CC teams can be vertical or hierarchical in nature; however, applying the idea of shared leadership may result in a more collaborative model in which all team members feel both the freedom and creativity to lead while being accountable for the outcomes.

PSYCHIATRISTS' ROLE IN PATIENT-CENTERED MEDICAL HOMES AND ACCOUNTABLE CARE ORGANIZATIONS

At the time of the writing of this chapter, the country was on the eve of a historic turning point in the delivery of health care services. The Patient Protection and Affordable Care Act was passed in 2010 by the administration of President Barack Obama, and the final implementation began on January 1, 2014, with millions of people gaining health insurance coverage. As mentioned in Chapter 1, psychiatrists have a unique role to play in these health care delivery systems, which have shown they can effectively improve the quality of care delivered while containing the escalating costs of treatment. In addition to improved outcomes, the reimbursement models of PCMHs and accountable care organizations offer solutions to the funding barriers that have heretofore limited the ability of teams, including psychiatrists, to get paid for much of the indirect work that goes into managing populations of chronically ill patients. With the improved care coordination and treatment required in these models, CC teams will be better positioned to address high utilizers of health care resources and help lower costs by treating a subset of medical conditions that are known contributors to this problem (Melek et al. 2013). The health care system of the future will value psychiatric expertise in containing costs rather than deplore the profession's ability to generate revenue in fee-for-service environments.

The National Committee for Quality Assurance (www.ncqa.org) has established levels of PCMHs with the highest designated as a level 3 on a scale of 1 to 3. Varying amounts of reimbursement will most likely be tied to PCMH levels, and many organizations are choosing to start at level 3. The 2014 National Committee for Quality Assurance standards requires utilizing evidence-based guideline care and tracking of chronic conditions and must include mental health (e.g., depression, anxiety, bipolar disorder, attention-deficit/hyperactivity disorder) or substance use disorders (e.g., illegal drug use, prescription drug addiction, alcoholism). PCMH Standard 5, Element B, factors 3 and 4, requires on-site integration of primary care and behavioral health; this is a "must pass" element for level 3 recognition. In addition, as a part of the Comprehensive Health Assessment (PCMH Standard 3, Element C), there is the requirement to utilize the U.S. Preventive Services Task Force screening guidelines for depression and to screen all adults and adolescents utilizing a standardized tool. The guideline goes on to include the statement "when staff-assisted support systems are in place to assure adequate diagnosis, effective treatment and follow-up" (www.uspreventiveservicestaskforce.org/3rduspstf/depression/).

The CC models presented in this book offer a valuable way to help organizations meet the criteria for PCMHs and provide a psychiatric workforce prepared to address the behavioral health needs of the populations served (Katon and Unützer 2011; Unützer et al. 2013). For example, the TEAMcare model represents the first evidence-based model where there is psychiatric consultation supporting the provision of effective care of multiple chronic medical conditions and depression (Katon et al. 2010). In this model, poorly controlled dyslipidemia, hypertension, and/or diabetes are treated alongside depression using evidence-based pharmacologic guidelines for each condition. In addition to the consultant psychiatrist, the team has a PCP consultant to perform regular caseload review, and recommendations are made for all conditions according to the health indicator data (such as HbA1c level) in the registry (see Table 3–2). Nurse care managers are part of the TEAMcare collaboration and provide patient education, brief interventions, and care coordination for the medical conditions as well as the depression treatment.

TABLE 3–2. TEAMcare summary report: example with joint consultant psychiatrist and primary care provider recommendations

PHQ BL	PHQ now	BP BL	BP now	LDL BL	LDL now	A1c BL	A1c now	Recommendations (PCP and psychiatric consultant input)
24	19	161/99	152/87	142	122	10.3	9.8	Schedule direct psychiatric evaluation, increase metformin
18	10	165/102	149/95	189	190	8.6	7.9	Increase fluoxetine, increase atorvastatin
14	9	201/117	189/100	123	130	11.2	8.6	Add amlodipine, increase insulin
13	2	156/96	135/84	108	99	9.9	5.8	Continue current treatment

Note. BL=baseline; BP=blood pressure; LDL=low-density lipoprotein; PCP=primary care provider; PHQ=Patient Health Questionnaire.

Participating in PCMHs will provide an opportunity for the consulting psychiatrist to sharpen his or her skills in general medical care and form collegial partnerships with PCP colleagues. By assisting in the detection and treatment of behavioral health conditions in PCMHs and accountable care organizations, psychiatrists bring a strong influence and opportunity for realizing the dream of the Patient Protection and Affordable Care Act and the triple aim in health care.

Psychiatrist Experience Working in TEAMcare Model

Anecdotally, after doing TEAMcare, when I supervise a collaborative depression care manager or do a psychiatric consult on a patient with type 2 diabetes, I make sure they have received guideline-level meds to lower blood sugar, blood pressure, and low-density lipoprotein cholesterol, and if they have these in poor control, I refer them back to their doctor with some recommendations like increasing metformin or other meds. The experience of cosupervising depression and diabetes with a PCP has helped me to be a lot more alert to medical disease control and adherence.

W.K., TEAMcare consulting psychiatrist, Washington

PRIMARY CARE PROVIDER–PSYCHIATRIST PARTNERSHIP

Integrated care provides an interesting opportunity for reciprocal partnerships between psychiatric providers and their primary care colleagues and is currently a source of much untapped potential. While the focus of Section I of this book ("Behavioral Health in Primary Care Settings") is on the consultant psychiatrist working in the primary care setting to support PCPs in the detection and treatment of behavioral health conditions, Section II ("Primary Care in Behavioral Health Settings") is devoted to improving the health status of the population with serious mental illness (SMI). In this scenario, PCPs and psychiatrists again form an alliance to implement models of care to improve health outcomes and contain costs in this historically high-cost medical group. The role of the psychiatrist is shifting from an independent practitioner providing mental health treatment in the isolation of the counseling and mental health center environment to one that includes the recognition that teams are needed to address the treatment of both mental and physical health concerns leading to health disparities in the population with SMI. In the behavioral health setting, PCPs not only provide direct care in some locations but also are available as consultants to psychiatric providers as they begin to assume greater oversight of all the medical care of patients (see Chapter 8, "Providing Primary Care in Behavioral Health Settings," and Chapter 9, "Behavioral Health Homes").

Some emerging experiences may help guide the establishment of these partnerships and the shifting role of psychiatrists from "consultant" in the primary care setting to providing more medical oversight in the behavioral health setting. Trust has been identified as crucial to the partnership and allows the dyad to work more effectively. The PCP has to trust that the psychiatrist is there to back him or her up in prescribing and treating more complex patients in primary care and to work to effectively sell the CC model to patients and staff. One clever PCP decided the best way to engage patients and introduce the BHP was to use the line "I have someone here who is an expert in problem solving to help you." Failure of the PCP to effectively prescribe for these disorders or sell the model to patients can lead to less than robust outcomes and compromise the system.

In the behavioral health environment, the reverse is true. Because of the patient's enduring relationship with the psychiatric provider, he or she may be able to do a good job of selling the need for primary care to patients with SMI, who often have a lack of perceived need for health care. Having a relationship with the PCP during this sales pitch can help facilitate this referral. Also, guiding PCPs in their approach to patients in the behavioral health settings can lead to better engagement and avoid overwhelming patients who have a long list of unmet health care needs. PCPs and psychiatric providers need to organize care so duplicative services are not occurring and to coordinate obtaining laboratory and other services. Table 3–3 describes some tips from PCPs and psychiatrists who have worked in various settings along the integration spectrum.

TABLE 3–3.   Tips for successful primary care provider–psychiatrist partnerships

---

Sense of *humor* is critical; "absurd things happen," and you need to appreciate this without getting bent out of shape.

Defensiveness on the part of either the primary care provider (PCP) or the psychiatrist does not work well.

Flexibility to change the work flow given the presenting issues is essential.

PCP willingness to work on *engagement* first is fundamental; therapeutic relationship between the PCP and patient is key.

Patience to bite off one piece of the to-do list at a time so treatment is not so daunting is required; meet the patient where they are.

Desire to be part of a *team* is crucial; lone ranger does not work well in this environment.

Willingness to share *leadership* roles is essential.

Source.   Excerpts from "Shared Space and Merging Cultures: The PCP-Psychiatrist Partnership" workshop, Institute on Psychiatric Services Meeting, Philadelphia, PA, 2013.

THE SUCCESSFUL CONSULTANT PSYCHIATRIST

It is important to choose a psychiatric consultant who is the "best fit" for these aforementioned roles on the CC team. Knowledge of the evidence base, core principles, and specific tasks for CC teams is important to maintain adherence to the model in order to achieve the best possible outcomes. This knowledge will be vital if the team begins to stray from the potential discomfort of practice change back to the more familiar stance of colocated care. Staying current with publications and advances in the field can provide teams with new insights on successful techniques and ideas for expansion to different populations and diagnostic groups. The ability to be flexible and adapt to the needs of the primary care environment allows the unique aspects of any given clinic, or the available community resources, to be incorporated into the model. The willingness to be available and interrupted by the on-site primary care team is crucial to allowing immediate input and adjustments to care to prevent delays in treatment. Managing concerns about liability for consultation on patients who have not been directly evaluated is important, and an understanding of this risk will be necessary for those considering these roles. Last, having some knowledge and skill in leading teams can help make the difference between a successful partnership and a failed endeavor since working around resistance and finding solutions is required in the inherently challenging task of merging the cultures of primary care and behavioral health.

CONCLUSION

The consulting psychiatrist has an array of important roles to play on collaborative care teams to help ensure meaningful clinical, operational, and financial outcomes. These roles range from direct patient evaluations, to caseload-based population management, to providing leadership and education to ensure positive team interactions and adherence to the model. Psychiatric involvement in PCMH initiatives will add considerable value and help bring about desperately needed changes in the management of multiple chronic conditions. Psychiatrists best suited for these roles will possess a select skill set and attitude that will lead to their successful participation and leadership on these teams.

REFERENCES

Bauer AM, Azzone V, Goldman HH, et al: Implementation of collaborative management at community-based primary care clinics: an evaluation. Psychiatr Serv 62(9):1047–1053, 2011

Cerimele JM, Chan YF, Chwastiak LA et al: Bipolar disorder in primary care: clinical characteristics of 740 primary care patients with bipolar disorder. Psychiatr Serv doi: 10.1176/appi.ps.201300374 April 15, 2014. http://ps.psychiatryonline.org/Article.aspx?ArticleID=1861987. Accessed May 23, 2014. [epub ahead of print]

Ernst C, Chrobot-Mason D: Boundary Spanning Leadership. Published in partnership with the Center for Creative Leadership. New York, McGraw-Hill, 2011

Katon W, Unützer J: Consultation psychiatry in the medical home and accountable care organizations: achieving the triple aim. Gen Hosp Psychiatry 33:305–310, 2011

Katon WJ, Lin EH, Von Korff M, et al: Collaborative care for patients with depression and chronic illnesses. N Engl J Med 363(27):2611–2620, 2010

Melek S, Norris D, Paulus J: Economic Impact of Integrated Medical-Behavioral Health: Implications for Psychiatry. American Psychiatric Association Report to the Ad Hoc Workgroup on Health Care Reform. Denver, CO, Milliman, 2013

Olick RS, Bergus GR: Malpractice liability for informal consultations. Fam Med 35(7):476–481, 2003

Pearce CL: The future of leadership: combining vertical and shared leadership to transform knowledge work. Academy of Management Perspectives 18(1):47–59, 2004

Unützer J, Katon W, Callahan CM, et al: Collaborative care management of late-life depression in the primary care setting. JAMA 288(22):2836–2845, 2002

Unützer J, Harbin H, Schoenbaum M, et al: The collaborative care model: an approach for integrating physical and mental health care in Medicaid health homes. Baltimore, MD, Health Home Information Resource Center, Center for Medicare & Medicaid Services, 2013

CHAPTER 4

 Child and Adolescent Psychiatry in Integrated Settings

Barry Sarvet, M.D.
Robert Hilt, M.D.

Pediatric primary care providers (PCPs) have a long history of promoting integrated care with a goal of providing a comprehensive care environment for families. The term *medical home* was, in fact, first utilized by the American Academy of Pediatrics back in 1967 and subsequently evolved as a concept over the following decades to the point where the patient-centered health care home is now widely embraced by all of primary care medicine (Sia et al. 2004). The passage of the Patient Protection and Affordable Care Act in 2010 has accelerated the adoption of integrated models of pediatric primary care as a strategy to improve the health of populations and the quality and affordability of health care services.

PCPs now find that they are being asked to manage high volumes of child behavioral health care needs. It has been reported that about 50% of pediatric office visits involve behavioral, emotional, developmental, psychosocial, and/or educational concerns, and about 75% of the children with psychiatric disorders are being brought to see a pediatric PCP (Martini et al. 2012). The overall role of pediatric primary care has been gradually shifting from a relative focus on managing acute infections and illness to a greater focus on managing chronic conditions, behavioral health disorders, and developmental disabilities (Tanner et al. 2009). For instance, between 1979 and 1996 psychosocial problems being treated by pediatric primary care increased by 275%, a trend that has continued to this day (Kelleher et al. 2000).

PEDIATRIC PRIMARY CARE ENVIRONMENT

PCPs enjoy many advantages over specialty behavioral health professionals when they provide child mental health care. Pediatric PCPs are highly familiar with normal child development and thus are good at recognizing deviation from normal. They typically have long-term treatment relationships and a high level of trust with their patients at the time mental health problems appear. Families typically experience far less stigma about bringing their children to primary rather than specialty psychiatric care, and their office locations are usually more convenient and accessible for families than those of child mental health specialists. However, there are many important challenges in providing behavioral health care services to children that collaborative care systems need to address (American Academy of Pediatrics Task Force on Mental Health 2007). These challenges can be summed up in three general categories: time, training, and teamwork.

Time is a challenge for addressing behavioral health concerns because it takes more than twice as much office time to address any behavioral health problem than a strictly medical problem (Meadows et al. 2011). Providers commonly report that even a single complicated behavioral health patient can negatively impact their office flow while they are regularly seeing 25–30 patients daily. Although office routines could simply be adjusted to schedule more time for behavioral health patients, financial concerns about this time commitment remain. Unlike outpatient psychiatry, pediatric practices typically operate with a very high overhead for items such as vaccine purchases and extensive nurse and clinical assistant staffing, which makes them quite sensitive to even small reimbursement pressures. In one national study, net billing code reimbursement for provider time spent on child behavior health appointments was found to be as much as 4 times less per minute than for medical-focused appointments (Meadows et al. 2011). This means that physician owners of practices have had financial reasons to resist increasing their practice's time dedicated to behavioral health concerns.

Training is a challenge because pediatric PCPs report a lack of knowledge about how to effectively and confidently manage mental health conditions (American Academy of Pediatrics Task Force on Mental Health 2007). Behavioral health issues are a leading cause of disability in children; they constitute around 20% of the chief complaints treated in outpatient pediatric practice and are a corollary concern in up to 50% of all office visits (Cassidy and Jellinek 1998; Gardner et al. 2000). However, only around 5% of the training time in pediatric residency is focused on behavioral health. Trainees receive 4 weeks of experience in developmental/behavioral pediatrics (where the focus is on developmental disabilities) and 4 weeks of experience in adolescent medicine (where depression and substance use are part of the focus) over the course of a

3-year pediatric residency (Accreditation Council for Graduate Medical Education 2012). Family medicine residencies do place a relatively stronger emphasis on behavioral health care throughout their training, but adult issues typically overshadow learning about child behavioral health. After residency is completed, providers might read or attend lectures about child mental health issues; however, research on medical education has shown this is a relatively ineffective way to gain skills that are put into practice (Clark 2006; Prober and Heath 2012). On-the-job training and problem-based learning experience are better ways to learn behavioral health treatment skills.

Teamwork in behavioral health diagnosis and treatment is particularly important because PCPs routinely report lacking specialists to discuss cases with, specialty resources to refer to, and referral sites that would provide feedback and share decision making with them (American Academy of Pediatrics Task Force on Mental Health 2007). With support, PCPs should be able to manage children in their practices with mild to moderate functional impairments from anxiety, depression, inattention/impulsivity, disruptive behavior/aggression, substance abuse, and learning difficulties (Foy et al. 2010).

MODELS OF INTEGRATED PSYCHIATRIC PRACTICE IN PEDIATRIC PRIMARY CARE

It could be argued that if psychiatry were fully integrated into pediatric primary care, it would be seamlessly interwoven into the process of care and not be recognizable as a separate function. During well-child visits for children of all ages, there would be thorough consideration of mental health status, and parents and children would be routinely educated about preventing and managing risk factors associated with mental health difficulties. For children with active mental health problems, definitive diagnoses would be made, and these concerns would be clearly identified and continuously managed in a care plan. Similar to any medical condition, a variety of ancillary and specialty care services would need to be coordinated within the care plan, and the patient's progress would be tracked with applicable outcome measures. The pediatrician would not be expected to know as much about psychiatric illness as a child and adolescent psychiatrist; however, the pediatric care team would have the knowledge and skill to make initial psychiatric diagnoses, to connect patients to appropriate community mental health resources, to prescribe and monitor routine psychiatric medications, and to assess clinical progress. Given the challenges of time, training, and teamwork described in the section "Pediatric Primary Care Environment," pediatric primary care practices need substantial resources in order to enable them to provide such an integrated service for children and families. Child and adolescent psychiatrists and other children's mental health experts are becoming more aware of this need, and some programmatic service delivery models for the provision of these functions to psychiatric teams have emerged (Keller and Sarvet 2013). Given the shortage of child and adolescent psychiatrists, new models that leverage their expertise are urgently needed.

Before consideration of these models, it is important to note that the *pediatric primary care team*, rather than a pediatrician, as the provider of pediatric primary care service has gained ascendancy in the context of health care reform in the United States. While the pediatrician, family physician, or pediatric nurse-practitioner leads this team in partnership with the patient and family, this team concept implicitly acknowledges that high-value pediatric primary care cannot be delivered at scale by one person and that one of the most important skills of a pediatric PCP is to be able to lead this group and to delegate certain tasks and responsibilities, prioritizing and coordinating the care while keeping track of the big picture with the assistance of health information technology (American Academy of Pediatrics Medical Home Initiatives for Children With Special Needs Project Advisory Committee 2004). Although colocation of behavioral health resources offers significant advantages, particularly in light of the well-described barriers to mental health referral from primary care settings, the primary care team is certainly not contained by the walls of the pediatric office setting. The success of integrated care models in pediatric settings is dependent on the degree to which the psychiatric resources are able to participate in the delivery of primary care service as full members of the primary care team.

Child Psychiatry Access Programs

Exemplified by the Massachusetts Child Psychiatry Access Project (MCPAP) and the Partnership Access Line at the University of Washington, child psychiatry access models have been spreading across the nation, currently represented in 24 states (National Network of Child Psychiatry Access Programs 2013, www.nncpap.org). In general, child psychiatry access programs (CPAPs) are designed to enhance the capacity of pediatric practices to integrate behavioral health into primary care service by providing pediatric PCPs with readily accessible informal and formal clinical consultation from a team of child and adolescent psychiatrists, care coordinators, and other clinical professionals working from a separate location. The informal consultation is most commonly provided via telephone but may also be delivered through other forms of electronic communication such as e-mail or televideo connection. The informal consultation is meant to provide continuous, rapid availability for any mental health question arising in primary care practice, no matter how trivial. Questions that require more extensive consideration result in expedited scheduling of a formal clinical consultation at an accessible location or by a telepsychiatry procedure for remote locations. Programs include experienced psychiatric care coordinators who are available to assist practices with referrals for psychotherapy and other necessary mental health services and to ensure that PCPs receive information about the services that have been arranged. PCPs utilizing this type of program over time experience improvement in their overall psychiatric knowledge and skill by having brief case-based educational experiences whenever they use the informal telephone consultation. The care coordination component of the program helps practices to establish linkages with the children's mental health service providers in their community, essential to their role in providing a medical home to their patients with psychiatric illness. Patients may be tracked in registries to ensure that follow-up appointments are kept and that no one "falls through the cracks" in the treatment and referral process. Programs may also offer additional clinical services, including brief psychotherapy and care coordination follow-up to offer further assistance to families with establishing treatment in the community.

Case Example: Use of Child Psychiatry Access Program

R.F. is a 14-year-old boy living in an extremely rural community with his Spanish-speaking mother. A few years ago he was functioning fairly well in school, but he now refuses to go to school on most days. He sleeps poorly, is often up pacing and talking to himself, and has become increasingly withdrawn. His outpatient therapist from the nearest mental health center diagnosed him with an anxiety disorder. His mother reports that the counseling he gets has not been helping, and she is hoping that the PCP could prescribe a medicine for anxiety. After meeting with R.F., the PCP suspects that there is more going on here than just anxiety. The PCP discusses the case with the consulting child and adolescent psychiatrist who is on call for the CPAP for their region, who agrees it would be unwise to initiate any medication until R.F.'s diagnosis is clearer. An expedited consultation is scheduled via telemedicine, and the patient is found to have a history and examination consistent with early-onset schizophrenia. Hospitalization is discussed but is declined by the family, and his current level of functioning is deemed not to meet involuntary commitment standards. Because the next available appointment for a community child and adolescent psychiatrist is more than 2 months away, the PCP and collaborating consultant work out an antipsychotic management plan for the patient that they will jointly monitor until the patient's care can be transferred into specialty care. During those next 2 months, there is frequent contact with the family and between the providers, and R.F.'s psychotic symptoms are successfully stabilized through the medication trial and parent coaching on managing his difficulties. By then, the patient's care has been transitioned to the local mental health clinic as a result of earlier referral by the CPAP care coordinator. The care coordinator ensures that the patient's family is aware of the appointment, provides the mental health clinic with records of the psychiatric treatment to date, and helps the parent to complete releases to enable communication between the clinic and the PCP, who will be continuing to monitor the patient's overall health status.

With psychiatric services provided from a remote location, CPAPs can support integration for multiple primary care practices over a large geographic area, extending scarce child psychiatrist resources to a larger population of patients. For these essentially on-demand programs to operate effectively, the primary care practices must be motivated to call for consultation; therefore, the programs must employ strategies to promote engagement in the model. Some of these strategies include providing outreach visits; organizing regional conferences; distributing resources such as newsletters and parent education materials; and employing clinical rating scales. Utilization tends to be reinforced through satisfactory experiences with the service, and as a result, the programs become incorporated into the busy primary care work flow. Successful implementations of this model have reported progressive growth in utilization over a period of 3–5 years (Hilt et al. 2013; Sarvet et al. 2010). Frequency of utilization, reflecting engagement of the primary care practices with the program, is a key indicator of program performance and should therefore be carefully monitored.

Growth of Knowledge of Primary Care Provider Over Time

Even though they are not physically here in my office, I have grown to consider the MCPAP team as part of my practice. I call them several times a day and find them to be indispensable in my daily work. Before this program was available, I found mental health issues in my practice to be quite overwhelming and felt that they should be someone else's job. With the help of MCPAP, I have come to feel that my practice is well equipped for this, and frankly, I think that it's quite appropriate for me to be dealing with these issues as part of kids' overall health care.

P.K., pediatrician, Massachusetts

Case Example: Supporting Interim Primary Care Provider Management of Complex Psychiatric Illness

G.R. is a 9-year-old boy, discharged a few weeks ago from a residential treatment facility in another state, brought to see his new PCP. His mother says that her son has five prescriptions that will all be running out tomorrow, and she needs to get them all refilled because "he is a mess if he doesn't get his meds." She says she called the facility's medication prescriber for a refill first and was told that because her son's treatment is now completed, mom needed to see a new provider for those refills. Their local mental health center has scheduled an intake screening in 2 weeks, and the soonest they might see a prescriber is more than a month from now. On exam in the office, G.R. does not seem to be having any behaviors that are atypical for a child his age, although he appears a bit sleepy. His current medications are lamotrigine 100 mg twice a day, sertraline 100 mg every morning, risperidone 1 mg every morning and 2 mg each evening, clonidine 0.4 mg every night, and osmotic-release oral system (OROS) methylphenidate 54 mg every morning. His mother reports that prior to his 5-month residential stay, he was having a lot of tantrums at home, which is not happening now. The PCP contacts the child and adolescent psychiatry consultant from their regional CPAP to talk through what to do next. She notes that she often does temporary refills of psychiatric medications but that this combination of five medications for a 9-year-old concerns her. The consultant acknowledges that this medication regimen is quite intensive for a prepubertal child and is associated with potential long-term medical risks; however, the consultant cautions the PCP that significant changes should be made only after a thorough review of the history and that any changes should be made cautiously and gradually. Supporting the interim management of G.R.'s treatment, the consultant advises the PCP about the dose ranges, potential side effects, and medical monitoring standards for these medications. As a result of the consultant's request for additional clinical history regarding the patient's functioning and behavioral observations, it is discovered that G.R. is experiencing moderate sedation every morning and having difficulty getting out of bed for school. After consideration of this history and the information provided by the consultant, the PCP decides to gradually reduce the dose of the bedtime clonidine and risperidone. At follow-up several days later, G.R.'s mother reports that he is no longer sedated and that his behavior is remaining stable. The care coordinator from the CPAP is able to secure an expedited intake for G.R., to be followed by a psychiatric nurse-practitioner appointment at the local mental health center within 6 weeks. In the meantime, the PCP has G.R. return for several follow-up visits in order to monitor his behavioral health status and appropriate medical parameters during this period.

Integrated Behavioral Health Providers in Pediatric Settings

The physical presence of a children's mental health clinician in a primary care practice is often a very desirable solution and is the cornerstone of models of integration exemplified by North Carolina's Primary Care Children's Mental Health Initiative (Williams et al. 2006). Because of workforce and cost considerations, the pediatric behavioral health provider (BHP) is usually a licensed clinical social worker or psychologist. When the schedule for this clinician has adequate time built in, it becomes possible for the child to receive a thorough evaluation of suspected mental health problems without significant barriers or delay. The immediate availability of the BHP allows the PCP to delegate the tasks of assessment and behavioral health care coordination and planning for the mental health problem to a specialist who is ordinarily more comfortable with these tasks. As long as the BHP functions as a full member of the primary care team, behavioral health care may be coordinated within the context of the child's overall health care. Successful models provide training to ensure that the clinical work is adapted to the needs of the primary care setting, which includes the BHP focusing primarily on clinical assessment and care coordination. BHPs may directly organize and support mental health screening initiatives in primary care practices, utilizing validated "broadband" instruments such as the Pediatric Symptom Checklist (Jellinek et al. 1988) as well as more focused instruments such as the Patient Health Questionnaire for Adolescents (PHQ-A; Johnson et al. 2002), the CRAFFT screening tool (a behavioral health screening tool used with children under 21 years at risk for alcohol and substance use; the acronym stands for key components: car, relax, alone, forget, friends, trouble; Knight et al. 2002), and the Screen for Child Anxiety Related Emotional Disorders (SCARED; Birmaher et al. 1997).

BHPs also frequently provide informal "curbside" consultation to PCPs and are often available for "warm handoffs," which allow the busy PCP to move on to the next exam room while the BHP completes an assessment of the behavioral health issues. BHPs also assist in the ongoing monitoring of identified mental health issues, utilizing assessment tools such as the PHQ-A and the Vanderbilt ADHD Diagnostic Parent Rating Scale (Wolraich et al. 2003). Because of space limitations, the pediatric setting is usually not conducive to the provision of conventional outpatient therapy; however, BHPs can provide brief problem-focused therapeutic intervention such as motivational interviewing, relaxation training, and mindfulness-based stress reduction, as well as psychoeducation and anticipatory guidance counseling for common behavioral problems. Some of these therapeutic interventions may be offered in a group setting. As members of the primary care team, BHPs document their work within a shared medical record.

The following actions are essential to anticipatory guidance counseling in pediatric primary care settings (adapted from S. Reuille-Dupont, LPC, Colorado, unpublished communication, September 2013):

1. Educating parents regarding normal social and emotional development
2. Training parents in basic behavior-modification principles: establishment of consistent expectations and structure, clear limit setting, praise, and positive reinforcement
3. Teaching strategies to enhance parent-child relationships
4. Teaching strategies to improve family cohesion and address sibling conflicts
5. Coaching parents on addressing bullying issues

6. Educating parents about impact of toxic stress and traumatic experiences
7. Helping parents become effective advocates for their children with regard to addressing special educational needs
8. Utilizing cognitive-behavioral principles to help parents manage mild manifestations of generalized anxiety, social anxiety, and separation anxiety
9. Helping to prepare children and parents for therapy referrals and educating them regarding what to expect
10. Providing stress management techniques: relaxation training and introduction to mindfulness-based stress reduction

Although it is ordinarily not possible for child and adolescent psychiatrists to have a continuous presence in a primary care practice and thereby function as BHPs, these models invariably require their involvement for clinical consultation on complex and high-risk patients and/or patients with treatment-refractory conditions as well as psychopharmacology consultation. Some systems utilize "circuit-riding" child psychiatrists who might be available to provide consultation regarding diagnostic clarification and/or psychopharmacology questions for a block of time on a weekly or monthly basis in each primary care practice. Others may pair a BHP model with a CPAP in order to fulfill these comprehensive needs.

Case Example: Helping Primary Care Providers Establish Accurate Diagnosis

B.L. is a 6-year-old girl presented with her mother to her PCP because of uncontrolled hyperactivity and oppositional behavior at home. A relative suggested that she might have attention-deficit/hyperactivity disorder (ADHD) and that her mother should ask the PCP to prescribe Ritalin. The PCP proposes that the BHP working within their office conduct a clinical evaluation and does a warm handoff with the parent and child; the BHP meets with the parent and child for 20 minutes to gather additional history. The clinician discovers that the symptoms of hyperactivity and oppositionality have been going on for several years. Specific descriptions of the behavior include general overarousal and anxiety, as well as quite intense tantrums triggered by frustration or any attempt at redirection. During tantrums, the child is verbally abusive to her mother, echoing specific phrases that her biological father used to say to her mother prior to their separation 3 years ago. B.L.'s mother is a single parent who reports that she suffered persistent domestic abuse from B.L.'s father, who had been diagnosed with bipolar disorder. She experienced depression during this period and did not believe that B.L. had witnessed all of this. The BHP briefly teaches B.L. a breathing exercise to help her with anxiety and schedules the mother and daughter for a second visit. At a second visit with the BHP, B.L.'s mother brings Vanderbilt rating scales that have been completed by B.L.'s mother as well as the child's teacher.

These indicate symptoms of hyperactivity and inattention at home but none at school. Further history and interview of the child reveal evidence of traumatic play in which she reenacted scenes of harassment and victimization between dolls. B.L. does not have significant behavioral issues at school, with the exception of some problems with peers in unstructured situations. Screening with the SCARED tool scores positive for anxiety. On the basis of her assessment, the BHP makes a preliminary diagnosis of posttraumatic stress disorder, advises the PCP that prescribing a psychostimulant is not indicated, educates B.L.'s mother about the diagnosis, develops a treatment plan that includes referral to trauma-informed psychotherapy at a community mental health agency, and connects B.L.'s mother to a local parent support group for women who have experienced domestic violence. B.L. is seen for one additional session by the BHP 4 weeks later to review progress and ensure that services are being provided in the community. The BHP educates the PCP about the patient's need for ongoing monitoring of social and emotional development on the basis of the diagnosis of posttraumatic stress disorder and about the elevated risk of bipolar disorder. These issues are noted in B.L.'s problem list and primary care plan.

Because neither the CPAP nor the BHP model has the capacity to deliver comprehensive mental health care within the primary care setting, primary care practices must build up strong collaborative relationships with mental health resources in the surrounding community. This may also include establishing linkages with BHPs practicing within school-based health centers, an increasingly important resource for reaching children with unmet mental health needs. Assistance with this development is a function of both models.

Case Example: Supporting Community Mental Health Surveillance Initiatives

D.S. is a 16-year-old girl seen for an annual history and physical by her PCP at the school-based health center. The practice routinely administers the PHQ-A screening instrument for adolescents. D.S. reports depressive symptoms of moderate severity (PHQ-A score of 16). D.S.'s mother reports that her grades were much lower than usual this past term and that she has been more withdrawn and irritable over the past 4 months. As usual for adolescents, the PCP meets privately with D.S. during the exam and talks with her briefly about some of the symptoms she has reported on the PHQ-A. D.S. admits that she has been feeling sad most of the time. She has lost interest in her classes and activities and feels that no one understands her. She denies suicidal ideation (score is 0 on the suicidality question #9 on the PHQ-A). The PCP tells D.S. and her mother that there is a likelihood that she is experiencing depression and recommends that she meet the BHP in their practice. The clinician is available to meet D.S. briefly at the end of the visit, instructs her in a behavioral activation exercise, and arranges for her to come back for an appointment several days later. Upon evaluation, the BHP finds that D.S. is suffering from a major depressive disorder that began about 6 months earlier after she experienced a painful breakup with her boyfriend. There is a family history of depression on her father's side of the family. The BHP carefully explores the issue of suicidality and finds that D.S. has, in fact, experienced some passing thoughts about there being no point in living, but D.S. denies any actual suicidal urges, plans, or intentions. In negotiating treatment options, the clinician discovers that D.S. and her family would prefer beginning with psychotherapy rather than medication. She lets them know that psychotherapy is a recommended initial treatment for moderate depression. She also educates them about the safety and effectiveness of selective serotonin reuptake inhibitor (SSRI) medication and informs them that this medication might be recommended by her PCP if her therapy does not result in improvement over the next 6 weeks. She also develops a safety plan with D.S. regarding what to do if she has any worsening of her suicidal thoughts. The clinician discusses her findings with the PCP, who makes the additional recommendation for D.S. to be screened for hypothyroidism. The BHP makes a referral for D.S. to see a local therapist for cognitive-behavioral therapy and arranges follow-up at the primary care practice on a monthly basis to repeat her PHQ-A and monitor progress. This is documented in the clinic chart.

EVIDENCE BASE AND EXPERIENCES WITH INTEGRATION MODELS IN PEDIATRIC PRIMARY CARE

Nearly all of the more than 79 randomized trials that have demonstrated advantages in collaborative or integrated mental health care systems have been specific to the treatment of adult patients (Unützer 2013). A large evidence disparity between adult and child research therefore exists despite there being a broad recognition within the health care community of the vast shortcomings of the current child mental health service system that must similarly be addressed. The reasons why there are comparatively far fewer collaborative care outcomes research studies completed with children are many, including the following: 1) for both regulatory and family reasons, enrollment of children into formal research studies tends to be a far more cumbersome process than with adults, and 2) children are a relatively smaller population than adults, placing a much smaller financial burden on the health care system as a whole than adults, and thus are less often targeted by federal research dollars aiming to redesign the mental health system.

There is, however, a fairly extensive literature documenting the need to provide mental health education for pediatric primary care and the need to provide better collaborative and integrative care structures between pediatric primary care and mental health services. Both the American Academy of Pediatrics and the American Academy of Child and Adolescent Psychiatry have proposed models and methods for improved specialty collaboration, because both specialties now accept this need for improved collaboration as a given (American Academy of Pediatrics Task Force on Mental Health 2007; Martini et al. 2012). Increasing the mental health specialist workforce alone is an incomplete solution, in part because families often resist engaging with a physically separated specialty mental health system. For instance, in one study, about 40% of children appropriately referred to specialty mental health by their PCP were found to never attend a single mental health specialist appointment, and about 70% of appropriately referred children failed to attend more than a single mental health appointment over the next 6 months (Rushton et al. 2002). The old model of simply making a referral to an available specialist often means the child receives inadequate treatment.

There are no controlled trials of what has been proposed as the ideal model of integrated care in children, in which both pediatric primary care and mental health specialty care have become fully merged and transformed into an integrated, patient- and family-centered practice within the same physical space. One care model for which at least some partial outcome reports are publicly available is the Community Care of North Carolina (CCNC) system, which is a long-standing statewide Medicaid care management system using provider networks focused on chronic illness care, case management and clinical support, and data feedback to treating physicians. Starting in 2010, the CCNC was expanded more specifically into the behavioral health arena by employing a team of psychiatrists, behavioral health coordinators, and pharmacists to help 1,400 primary care practices to better deliver care for mild to moderate behavioral health disorders in both adults and children. This enhanced system provides education and enhanced communication between primary care and specialty care and in many locations will utilize a BHP colocated in the practice to provide enhanced screening and brief treatment (www.communitycarenc.org). It has been reported that the overall CCNC care coordination system has had significantly reduced overall costs of care and reduced emergency department utilization for children; however, outcome data specific to CCNC's more recent behavioral health coordination and colocated mental health providers are not yet available (Cosway et al. 2011; Treo Solutions 2012).

Similarly, the far more common practice of colocated child mental health specialists, such as child psychiatrists or licensed therapists, physically within a primary care practice without a formalized integration and care management assistance system lacks child-specific research evidence to show there are additional clinical benefits resulting from this colocation. The commonly theorized benefit of colocation is that this will decrease patient barriers to accepting and following through on a "warm handoff" mental health referral (i.e., to decrease no-show rates), but no data are available to show that this actually happens with children and families.

A system that provides for in-office master's-level care managers who screen, triage, provide psychoeducation for families, provide short-term cognitive-behavioral treatment, and monitor outcomes has, however, been studied and has been shown to yield greater outcome benefits in children (Kolko et al. 2012). This doctor-office collaborative care (DOCC) system also provides the clinical team with access to a skilled child psychiatrist for case consultation on children requiring intervention. The active comparison group in this study was *enhanced usual care*, in which the other children identified as having possible mental health concerns through the externalizing subscale of an abbreviated version of the Pediatric Symptom Checklist (Gardner et al. 1999) received care manager–delivered psychoeducation about their disorders and up to three personally tailored referral options. DOCC for externalizing behavior problems was found to have superior clinical outcomes in Vanderbilt ADHD Diagnostic Parent Rating Scale subscores for hyperactivity/impulsivity, overall ADHD symptoms, disruptive behavior, anxiety/depression, and conduct symptoms and on the Clinical Global Impression scale (61% improved vs. 0% from enhanced usual care). Both pediatricians and parents were highly satisfied with the DOCC system. The degree of investment over 6 months of active intervention for this result was that the care manager invested about 19 hours per child, mostly providing therapy, and PCPs invested a total of 1 hour per child (Kolko et al. 2012). An additional recent investigation utilized the DOCC design to deliver in-office evidence-based interventions for ADHD and anxiety problems and compared outcomes with enhanced usual care. This in-office active intervention was found to yield higher rates of treatment initiation and completion, more improvement in behavior problems, more improvement in hyperactivity and internalizing problems, reduced parental stress, and more consumer satisfaction (Kolko et al. 2014)

Another version of counseling services offered without a referral within pediatric medical offices has been studied for children and found to provide benefits. The Positive Parenting Program, "Triple P," is a multilevel intervention approach within primary care designed to deliver behavior management training to families in an easily accessed format that can rely on office nurses trained to deliver behavioral assistance, rather than licensed clinical therapists, to parents. Studies of Triple P found that a total of three or four nurse-run behavior management training sessions with parents led to reduced child behavior problems, reduced dysfunctional parenting, and reduced parental anxiety and stress, results that were largely maintained through a 6-month follow-up (Turner and Sanders 2006). For health system design, this was encouraging because, as opposed to needing to newly employ an in-office therapist, virtually every primary care office already employs a nurse who could conceivably receive such training. Predictors of office clinician success in the real-world delivery of primary care Triple P were higher nurse-reported self-efficacy after receiving program training and nurses reaching a belief that the program would offer their office an advantage over current office practices (Turner et al. 2011).

Pediatric medical practitioners would like to correctly identify clinical mental health problems and connect children and families to effective care, but this does not mean they are all interested in becoming the active providers of behavioral counseling for their patients (Taliaferro et al. 2013). This has led to an increasing interest in whether remotely delivered therapy services that are recommended and directed by the PCP could also be effective. Toward that end, multiple studies have now shown that online support and self-help readings on behavior management prescribed by the child's PCP can have equally significant and rapid treatment impacts compared with therapist-level delivered services (Lavigne et al. 2008; Sanders et al. 2012). Therefore, a parent who has been sufficiently motivated by their PCP to make a change in how he or she manages his or her child's behaviors can often do so without the help of an in-office therapist. However, for other child mental health problems, such as depression and anxiety, that are not so greatly reliant on changing parenting practices, this bibliotherapy approach has not been shown to be effective for children.

Other forms of remote specialty consultation and collaboration in child mental health have increased significantly in popularity over the years. This rise in popularity of televideo services is due to inadequate access to child mental health specialty services across the country. Notably, a recent workforce study indicated that there are 8.6 child and adolescent psychiatrists per 100,000 overall population and that they are poorly distributed, resulting in no local child and adolescent psychiatry availability in many large areas (Thomas and Holzer 2006). Furthermore, in rural areas where practice sizes are small, a colocated mental health specialist support service may not make sense either financially or per work flow volumes. Televideo psychiatric care provision and consultation has therefore been studied in multiple ways. Telemedicine provision of child psychiatry consultation with developmentally disabled children has been found to enable detection of unrecognized mental health conditions, to lead to changes in psychiatric medications, and to be associated with clinical improvement over time (Szeftel et al. 2012). Telemedicine appointments have been found to have high levels of satisfaction for children, parents, and PCPs that are sustained through return visits as well. Other televideo appointment outcomes include increased goal achievement for children in detention facilities and varying degrees of reported outcome improvements over care as usual across the available studies (Myers et al. 2011).

Telephone-based consultation care supports have similarly been designed to yield an enhanced, collaborative care practice environment. Part of the appeal of telephone-based collaboration is the relatively minimal infrastructure investment (i.e., no need to occupy clinical space in PCP offices, to redesign electronic medical records, or to physically move a child mental health specialist into an underserved location), and all providers in a state can immediately receive access to skilled child mental health consultation and collaboration support. These consultation systems work by encouraging PCPs to call a child psychiatrist on the consultation team who will be able to discuss in the moment any evaluation or treatment question that the PCP may have, backed up by both available care coordination and the ability of consultants to see children for an appointment when desired by the PCP. Provider self-report of benefit from consultations with the MCPAP system found that telephone consultations increase PCP self-reported ability to meet the psychiatric needs of their patients (from a baseline of 8% up to 63% of the time) and yielded consultations that were reported as clinically helpful by 91% of enrolled PCPs. Consultation requests included a need for diagnostic clarification, treatment recommendations, and questions regarding psychiatric medications. For 24% of MCPAP consultations, the PCP was noted to retain primary responsibility for treatment (Sarvet et al. 2010).

The similar Partnership Access Line telephone consultation service based in Seattle, Washington, had comparable findings to MCPAP regarding PCP satisfaction and gains in PCP mental health treatment skills. Notably, however, in the rural communities covered by this program, the provision of face-to-face consultations for eligible children via televideo was one-third as frequent, and the rural PCPs were much more likely to retain primary management of mental health care (Hilt et al. 2013; Sarvet et al. 2010). Patient outcomes from telephone-based consultation service systems are difficult to measure because telephone consulting teams generally do not establish direct treatment relationships with their patients. However, in one analysis, payment claims for psychotherapy appointments increased after a consultation call (i.e., a 130% increase for foster children), and the PCP prescribing of SSRI and ADHD medications increased after a consultation call but without increases in medication costs. This cost containment was attributed to the discussion of when generic medications are appropriate by the consultant psychiatrist (Hilt et al. 2013).

ADULT PSYCHIATRISTS CONSULTING IN PEDIATRIC PRIMARY CARE: UNIQUE ATTRIBUTES OF CHILD MENTAL HEALTH TO CONSIDER

In areas of the United States in which child and adolescent psychiatrists are unavailable, adult psychiatrists are frequently called on to support collaborative care in pediatric primary care. The old adage that "children are not miniature adults" is pertinent; adult psychiatrists may encounter significant challenges in extending the focus of their practice from adult medicine to pediatric primary care. The following considerations may also be useful to administrative psychiatrists involved in planning and oversight of collaborative care programs where psychiatrists trained in adult care are asked to provide care in areas where child and adolescent psychiatrists are not available to provide this consultation service.

Mental Health Screening in Pediatric Settings

A broad variety of mental health conditions are prevalent in the pediatric population. Because of the dramatic developmental transformations occurring throughout the age range of pediatric patients, integrated practices must utilize different strategies for children of different ages. During infancy, one of the most important mental health issues needing to be identified is parental postpartum depression. Pediatric PCPs are well positioned to engage new parents in discussions regarding the importance of their own mental health and well-being to the health of the child. In this context, PCPs may utilize tools such as the Edinburgh Postnatal Depression Scale (Cox et al. 1987). During early childhood (ages 0–4), screening for atypical or delayed communication and social/emotional development is particularly pertinent, and tools such as the Ages & Stages Questionnaires tool (Bricker and Squires 1999) are commonly used by pediatricians. The feasibility of using the Parents' Evaluation of Developmental Status screening instrument in primary care has been demonstrated (Schonwald et al. 2009). The Modified Checklist for Autism in Toddlers screening instrument has also been demonstrated to be quite useful in the primary care setting (Robins 2008). Some of the most common mental health conditions occurring in young school-age children include anxiety disorders and disruptive behavior disorders (such as ADHD and oppositional defiant disorder). Older children and adolescents need to be screened for depression and substance use disorders. Broad screening instruments such as the Pediatric Symptom Checklist are useful for such general mental health screening in primary care (Jellinek et al. 1988). More specific instruments targeting depression (PHQ-A; Johnson et al. 2002) and substance abuse (CRAFFT; Knight et al. 2002) should be utilized for adolescents. The SCARED screening instrument, mentioned in the section "Integrated Behavioral Health Providers in Pediatric Settings," can be helpful in detecting and following treatment response for anxiety disorders.

Working With Parents

Positive engagement with parents is a fundamental aspect of behavioral health service delivery in the pediatric setting. Young children are totally dependent upon their parents, and parents continue to have a profound influence on a child's development and adaptation through adolescence and young adulthood. Regardless of any adverse influences that are discovered or inferred, parents remain the most important agent of change in any treatment plan with young people. It therefore behooves clinicians to focus on areas of parental strength and to develop an alliance with them based on mutual respect. In the context of such an alliance, the parent will be much more likely to be receptive to the recommendations, psychoeducation, and therapeutic intervention that can be provided in the primary care setting.

BHPs in pediatric settings also need to consider family dynamics in the assessment of mental health presentations. For example, the behavioral problems of a child may be functioning to regulate conflicts in the parents' marital relationship, such as creating a conflict that distracts or derails parental conflicts. Consequently, it is important for BHPs and consulting psychiatrists to have an understanding of the family context of symptoms. Pediatric PCPs may be well aware of these contextual issues based on their longitudinal relationship with child and family.

Parent Experience of Integrated Care

I won't have to make so many appointments. We can all touch base at once and get a full picture at the same time. Any problems can be taken care of right then and there with some very knowledgeable people. I have a very positive feeling. The doctors are always so kind. They take the time to see what the kids are like, what's going on with them. They're not just asking me the questions. They're actually listening to the children and getting feedback from them.

Parent in integrated care setting, Colorado (McCrimmon 2012)

Developmental Context

At times, children's mental health symptoms are directly caused by developmental delays. For example, children with receptive and expressive language delays may develop negative behaviors stemming from frustration in communication. Conversely, psychiatric illnesses interfere with normative developmental experiences and frequently are associated with delays in social and emotional development. Furthermore, psychiatric symptoms must be gauged in relation to normative development. For example, preschool children cannot be expected to sit still and sustain attention as well as older children;

therefore, the assessment of difficulties in these areas when considering a diagnosis of ADHD must be made in comparison to age-specific norms. Because pediatricians see countless typical children at all ages, they often have a finely tuned ability to judge whether a symptom is significant for a given child. Clinicians who have not worked in a primary care setting may have much less exposure to children with normal development, so they would be wise to take cues from the pediatrician in considering the developmental context of symptoms. In this respect, the pediatric PCP's knowledge of the patient's development may nicely complement the general psychiatrist's knowledge of psychopathology.

Child-Serving Systems

There are a variety of social systems that have a profound influence on the lives of children. The educational system is perhaps the most important of these systems. Teachers are an important source of history for the assessment of psychiatric symptoms, and they, in turn, may want insight into the child's mental health issues in order to mitigate impacts on the child's educational experience. The BHP frequently needs to communicate with school personnel in order to have a complete understanding of the child's functioning, to provide consultation regarding the educational plan, and at times to advocate on behalf of the child. Other child-serving systems that need to be considered by integrated clinicians within the primary care team include the child welfare system and the juvenile justice system, each of which may have authority over the child. Each of these latter systems is a branch of state government, and their policies are determined by state regulations. Nonetheless, those primary care practices involved in assessing and coordinating mental health care for children must establish good lines of communication with caseworkers from these systems in order to fully understand the child's circumstances as well as to help these systems to consider the child's mental health needs in planning.

Long-Term Effects of Trauma and Adverse Childhood Experiences

There is a substantial body of evidence that childhood trauma and other adverse childhood experiences have been causally associated with significant long-term health problems and premature death in adulthood (Felitti et al. 1998; Shonkoff and Phillips 2000). Adult medical providers typically see these consequences after they have become established as chronic health problems over many years. Pediatric PCPs have a unique opportunity to address these issues before these chronic health issues emerge (Garner et al. 2012). Consequently, an important aspect of integrated pediatric practice is to prevent and mitigate the effects of these experiences. Pediatric BHPs have a critical role in helping a primary care team to improve their performance in detecting when children have been affected by adverse experiences, in educating parents about the impact of these experiences, and in applying psychosocial interventions such as child trauma-focused therapies in order to help children to recover from them.

Pediatric Psychopharmacology Practice in Primary Care

The use of psychiatric medication is rarely recommended as a sole intervention in the treatment of childhood psychiatric illnesses. For example, medications are often considered adjuncts to more primary interventions such as cognitive-behavioral therapy for anxiety disorders. For ADHD, although psychostimulant medication is frequently recommended as an ongoing treatment throughout the course of the condition, this treatment is ideally combined with various types of psychosocial intervention aimed at improving impulse control, problem solving, organizational skills, and self-esteem. Combined medication and psychotherapy is also a frequent standard of treatment for pediatric mood disorders.

Classes of medications commonly prescribed by pediatric PCPs include SSRIs, psychostimulants, α_2-agonists, and atomoxetine. Consequently, with consultation from collaborating psychiatrists, pediatric PCPs are well positioned to provide the psychiatric medication component of treatment for ADHD, anxiety disorders, and depression. For patients with more complex psychiatric medication needs such as treatment-refractory depression, bipolar disorder, and psychotic illnesses, patients are ordinarily triaged to the care of child and adolescent psychiatrists; however, with the help of CPAPs, PCPs may prescribe for these patients for an interim period while referrals are being arranged. The document "Primary Care Principles for Child Mental Health, version 4.0," published online by the Partnership Access Line in Seattle, Washington (Hilt 2013), contains practical guidelines including dosage and monitoring recommendations for the use of psychiatric medications in the pediatric primary setting.

DEVELOPING AN INTEGRATED PEDIATRIC BEHAVIORAL HEALTH WORKFORCE

Pediatric Behavioral Health Providers

Although integrated pediatric behavioral health care is an emerging field, it is projected that a relatively large workforce will be needed to meet the needs of an extensive pediatric primary care health system throughout the

United States (Blount and Miller 2009). The role of an integrated pediatric BHP is quite different from that of a conventional outpatient clinician. He or she must be a generalist, with a comprehensive scope of clinical practice matching that of the pediatric practice, and must be comfortable working with children of all ages (from 0 to 22) and the widest range of clinical presentations. Because integrated child behavioral health encompasses prevention, the BHP sees patients with subclinical or preclinical presentations not meeting formal diagnostic criteria for a mental illness. Pediatric BHPs generally need a substantial level of confidence and maturity of clinical skill, enabling them to be teachers of pediatric medical providers.

Working at the interface of pediatrics and behavioral health, BHPs need to learn the language of pediatrics, become familiar with pediatric physical health problems and developmental syndromes and their treatment, and become comfortable working with sick children and their families. This may include working with children who are acutely anxious about medical procedures and providing time-limited therapy to address pain management or obesity. Mastery of the existing knowledge base regarding the emotional consequences of physical illness on the child and family is necessary.

Psychotherapeutic skills especially suited for integrated care include cognitive-behavioral therapy for anxiety, motivational interviewing for modifying health risk behavior, parent behavior management skill training approaches, mindfulness-based stress reduction techniques, and crisis management (see anticipatory guidance counseling points in "Integrated Behavioral Health Providers in Pediatric Settings" section). It is also very helpful for clinicians to have group therapy skills, which may be useful in group medical visits.

Two of the more important aptitudes for BHPs to have are flexibility and tolerance for a lack of control over their practice. They should expect to work in settings that are not designed specifically for mental health work, such as medical examination rooms. Mental health practitioners in current care systems often prefer to have tight control over time, with sessions starting and ending at precise times. In pediatric settings, visits are often unplanned and squeezed in. Patients may be double- or triple-booked, with medical providers moving from room to room. Similarly, mental health encounters are frequently unplanned, and the clinical work must be adapted for brief sessions.

Pediatric Behavioral Health Provider Experience

My experience as an integrated care provider is twofold with patients. On one hand it is a phenomenal way to provide health care; on the other, it presents some difficulties. In the BHP role I found my job to be less creative in some ways and more in others. Often the topics I covered were redundant and routine (e.g., bedtime, teeth brushing, potty training, and social-emotional development). The model of therapy was much more directive than a therapist may be used to or prepared for. This change in hats requires the therapist to be comfortable giving direction and asking difficult questions from an early point in the relationship and to be prepared for any number of answers/questions that may arise. The therapist must creatively work within patient boundaries while being prepared for whatever arises. In integrated care, the patient is often presenting for a physical health issue and may not plan to discuss social/emotional health until a screening tool or inquiry brings it to the surface. The therapist must be prepared to deal with whatever arises and have interventions for safety and containment in limited amounts of time, sometimes as short as 5 minutes. This may be difficult for the therapist trained to allow time to bring forward issues that need to be addressed and time to contain them in a more complete way. A necessary tool is the therapist's ability to allow the psychological work to be incomplete as the patient leaves the office and to help the client to be OK with this, as well. As is often the case, psychological work takes time and may not be complete in each session; however, the fast pace of a Western medicine office creates a new urgency and spin on how to "wrap a client up."

S.D., BHP, integrated pediatric practice, Colorado

Child and Adolescent Psychiatrists

Working collaboratively with pediatric PCPs within integrated models of care delivery requires a distinct skill set and clinical practice style. Telephone consultation regarding patients who have not been directly evaluated is challenging for many psychiatrists, who are relatively uncomfortable with uncertainty and ambiguity. It is important for the child and adolescent psychiatrist to consider the telephone consultation to be educational in nature. The telephone consultant is not treating the patient by "remote control"; rather, he or she is teaching the PCP about clinical assessment and best practice standards. Teaching points must be delivered concisely and efficiently. The telephone consultation is not in any way comprehensive, yet the consultant must help the PCP to be alert to potential clinical risks. The telephone consultant must be able to focus in on the central question posed by the PCP but also address questions that the PCP may not know to ask. Finally, it is quite important for the telephone consultant to provide a satisfactory interaction in order to build engagement with the PCP through subsequent calls over time. In the authors' experience, aptitudes for this type of work include a strong interest in children's mental health problem prevention and access to care, collaborating with other medical providers, valuing practicality over certainty, flexibility, and a relatively low need for control. There also needs to be a comfort level around liability for providing informal consultations that do not involve direct evaluation of the child (see Chapter 5, "Risk Management and Liability Issues in Integrated Care"). One study by Knutson et al. (2014) demonstrated no instances of medical malpractice suits in more than 20,000 telephone consultations.

A Child Psychiatrist's Experience With Integrated Care Teams

Integrated care is an important advancement in the delivery of services to children and teens. It complements other methods of treatment through creating opportunities that reach a broader range of children with mental health and psychosocial needs. The team-oriented approach allows for more comprehensive treatment of children, as we are drawing on the expertise of individuals across disciplines. As a child and adolescent psychiatrist, I find this work very rewarding and strongly support the expansion of integrated care.

M.F., child and adolescent psychiatrist, Colorado

Pediatric Primary Care Providers

Variability in the utilization of CPAPs belies the broad range in the degree of interest among pediatric PCPs in incorporating mental health into their practice. As a matter of policy, organized pediatrics has fully embraced the need for incorporating mental health in pediatric primary care (American Academy of Pediatrics Task Force on Mental Health 2007; Foy et al. 2010); however, a lack of training and an accumulation of negative experiences have soured the perspective of some pediatricians. Nonetheless, pediatricians working in integrated models of practice are discovering that addressing mental health issues may be quite rewarding. Engagement with collaborating mental health professionals and programmatic strategies to incorporate team members within the practice able to perform the more time-intensive aspects of integrated mental health service delivery appear to be essential factors contributing to the adoption of integrated care by pediatric PCPs.

A Pediatrician's Experience With Integrated Care

Having practiced pediatric medicine for the past 16 years in multiple settings—from academic medicine at a large university-based tertiary care setting, to public health with the U.S. Public Health Service, to fee-for-service private practice—I feel that working in the integrated care setting is by far the most satisfying experience, for both the providers and the patients. I often hear from patients that they love being cared for by a team of professionals. They report feeling valued and that they feel that the quality of care they experience is the highest they have ever received. As a provider, it is satisfying to work in such a collaborative environment. It is seamless to address the whole patient as we have all the resources at our fingertips to be able to serve our patients whatever their needs may be. Ultimately, having all their physical and mental health needs addressed will lead to better overall health for the patient in the long run.

K.R., pediatrician, school-based health center, Colorado

RESIDENT/FELLOW CHILD AND ADOLESCENT TRAINING IN INTEGRATED CARE

Because models of integrated child behavioral health care are actively changing and evolving, this creates some challenges for identifying what specific content psychiatric residents and child psychiatry fellows will need to learn about integrated care for children. Despite the inherent challenge of teaching a continually evolving content, the fact that there are major changes under way in our health system is of primary importance to psychiatric trainees, and thus it is well worth integrating models of integrated care into curricula. Specific educational materials on integrated care useful for this effort can be drawn from resources such as this book, from federal entities such as the Substance Abuse and Mental Health Services Administration–Center for Integrated Health Solutions and the Center for Medicaid & Medicare Services, and from professional organizations such as the American Psychiatric Association and the American Academy of Child and Adolescent Psychiatry. In addition, a model psychiatric residency experience in integrated care is available on the Advancing Integrated Mental Health Solutions Center Web site and is described in more detail in Chapter 6 ("Training Psychiatrists for Integrated Care").

Every psychiatry resident would benefit from learning about the reasons for integrating care, the primary care experience, the basic principles of integration, and examples of integration models he or she might encounter or work with. Therefore, the following are suggested learning objectives for residents (more information is provided in Chapter 6):

1. **Learning the reasons for integrated care:** Didactic lectures that describe the clinical and business case for integrated care and teaching residents the public health argument for why integrated care is needed are essential. Some exposure to health services research can be helpful, which might include the challenges payers and health systems may have in measuring outcomes in community and integrated care settings. It would also be pertinent to provide information for residents about the local care system so they can gain an understanding of where most children with mental health problems are getting their care and who is prescribing the psychotropic medications.

2. **Learning about and experiencing primary care:** Didactic lectures about how one could work collaboratively with primary care, accompanied by psychiatric trainees getting experiences with pediatric clinical settings and the pediatric primary care perspective on mental health care, are crucial. Experience of pediatric primary care settings might come via arranged time in a pediatric continuity care clinic, scheduled collaborative office rounds, or joint case conferences. The American Academy of Pediatrics and American Academy of Child and Adolescent Psychiatry created a collaborative office rounds model in which pediatric residents have a joint case seminar with child psychiatry residents (Knight and DeMaso 1999).

3. **Learning current models of integrated care delivery:** A didactic description of integrated care models, coupled with residents getting experiences in integrated care delivery, is key. Teaching the core principles of effective collaborative care (see Chapter 1, "Evidence Base and Core Principles") can be a useful guide to understanding program elements. If there are local integrated care programs, such as those described in this chapter, getting residents some experiential time with these programs would be valuable. Another possibility is creating rotations in which psychiatric residents work collaboratively with pediatric primary care colleagues at their institution or even share ongoing continuity clinic cases with pediatric residents (Burkey et al. 2014).

CONCLUSION

Integrated models of pediatric primary care practice incorporating collaborative mental health professionals have been spreading throughout the United States in response to growing concerns regarding poor access to care and the need to improve the quality and efficiency of health care delivery. These models allow leveraging of limited child and adolescent psychiatric expertise by delivering psychiatric consultation and care coordination from a remote location as well as the embedding of pediatric BHPs as members of the primary care team on location within pediatric practices. These models have demonstrated preliminary evidence of feasibility and clinical effectiveness. There are significant differences in the needs of children compared to the needs of adults that must be addressed in the provision of integrated care. To support the further development of this field, significant attention needs to be given to workforce development through training of existing mental health professionals as well as residency training for the coming generation of psychiatrists.

REFERENCES

Accreditation Council for Graduate Medical Education: ACGME Program Requirements for Graduate Medical Education in Pediatrics. Chicago, IL, Accreditation Council for Graduate Medical Education, 2012. Available at: http://www.acgme.org/acgmeweb/Portals/0/PFAssets/2013-PR-FAQ-PIF/320_pediatrics_07012013.pdf. Accessed September 16, 2013.

American Academy of Pediatrics Medical Home Initiatives for Children With Special Needs Project Advisory Committee: Policy statement: organizational principles to guide and define the child health care system and/or improve the health of all children. Pediatrics 113 (5 suppl):1545–1547, 2004

American Academy of Pediatrics Task Force on Mental Health: Strategies for System Change in Children's Mental Health: A Chapter Action Kit. Elk Grove, IL, American Academy of Pediatrics, 2007

Birmaher B, Khetarpal S, Brent D, et al: The Screen for Child Anxiety Related Emotional Disorders (SCARED): scale construction and psychometric characteristics. J Am Acad Child Adolesc Psychiatry 36(4):545–553, 1997

Blount FA, Miller BF: Addressing the workforce crisis in integrated primary care. J Clin Psychol Med Settings 16(1):113–119, 2009

Bricker D, Squires J: Ages & Stages Questionnaires: A Parent-Completed, Child Monitoring System, 2nd Edition. Baltimore, MD, Paul H Brookes, 1999

Burkey MD, Kaye DL, Frosch E: Training in integrated mental health-primary care models: a national survey of child psychiatry program directors. Acad Psychiatry. May 7, 2014. Accessed May 26, 2014. [Epub ahead of print]

Cassidy L, Jellinek M: Approaches to recognition and management of childhood psychiatric disorders in pediatric primary care. Pediatr Clin North Am 45:1037–1052, 1998

Clark CE: Problem-based learning: how do the outcomes compare with traditional teaching? Br J Gen Pract 56:722–723, 2006

Cosway R, Girod C, Abbott B: Analysis of Community Care of North Carolina Cost Savings. Denver, CO, Milliman, 2011

Cox JL, Holden J, Sagovsky R: Detection of postnatal depression: development of the 10-item Edinburgh Postnatal Depression Scale. Br J Psychiatry 150:782–786, 1987

Felitti VJ, Anda RF, Nordenburg D: Relationship of childhood abuse and household dysfunction to many of the leading causes of death in adults. Am J Prev Med 14(4):245–258, 1998

Foy JM, Kelleher KJ, Laraque D, et al: Enhancing pediatric mental health care: strategies for preparing a primary care practice. Pediatrics 125 (suppl 3):S87–S108, 2010

Gardner W, Murphy M, Childs G, et al: The PSC-17: a brief pediatric symptom checklist including psychosocial problem subscales: a report from PROS and ASPN. Ambulatory Child Health 5:225–236, 1999

Gardner W, Kelleher KJ, Wasserman R, et al: Primary care treatment of pediatric psychosocial problems: a study from pediatric research in office settings and Ambulatory Sentinel Practice Network. Pediatrics 106(4):E44, 2000

Garner AS, Shonkoff JP, Siegel BS, et al: American Academy of Pediatrics policy statement: early childhood adversity, toxic stress, and the role of the pediatrician: translating developmental science into lifelong health. Pediatrics 129(1):E224–E231, 2012

Hilt R: Primary Care Principles for Child Mental Health, Version 4.0, 2013. Available at: http://www.palforkids.org/docs/Care_Guide/Care_Guide_4.0_WA_Online_Version.pdf. Accessed December 8, 2013.

Hilt RJ, Romaire MA, McDonell MG, et al: Partnership Access Line: evaluating a consult program in Washington State. JAMA Pediatr 167(2):162–168, 2013

Jellinek MS, Murphy JM, Robinson J, et al: The Pediatric Symptom Checklist: screening school-age children for psychosocial dysfunction. J Pediatr 112:201–209, 1988

Johnson JG, Harris ES, Spitzer RL, et al: The Patient Health Questionnaire for adolescents: validation of an instrument for the assessment of mental disorders among adolescent primary care patients. J Adolesc Health 30(3):196–204, 2002

Kelleher KJ, McInerny TK, Gardner WP, et al: Increasing identification of psychosocial problems: 1979–1996. Pediatrics 105(6):1313–1321, 2000

Keller D, Sarvet B: Is there a psychiatrist in the house? Integrating child psychiatry into the pediatric medical home. J Am Acad Child Adolesc Psychiatry 52(1):3–5, 2013

Knight JR, DeMaso D: Collaborations Essentials for Psychiatry and Pediatric Residents: Working Together to Treat the Child. Special seminar preceding the annual meeting of the American Academy of Child and Adolescent Psychiatry, Chicago, IL, 1999

Knight JR, Sherritt L, Harris SK, et al: Validity of the CRAFFT substance abuse screening test among adolescent clinic patients. Arch Pediatr Adolesc Med 156:607–614, 2002

Knutson KH, Wei MH, Straus JH, et al: Medico-legal risk associated with pediatric mental health telephone consultation programs. Adm Policy Ment Health 41(2):215–219, 2014

Kolko DJ, Campo JV, Kilbourne AM, et al: Doctor-office collaborative care for pediatric behavioral problems: a preliminary clinical trial. Arch Pediatr Adolesc Med 166(3):224–231, 2012

Kolko DJ, Campo J, Kilbourne AM, et al: Collaborative care outcomes for pediatric behavioral health problems: a cluster randomized trial. Pediatrics 133:e981–e992, 2014

Lavigne JV, Lebailly SA, Gouze KR, et al: Treating oppositional defiant disorder in primary care: a comparison of three models. J Pediatr Psychol 33(5):449–461, 2008

Martini R, Hilt R, Marx L, et al: Best principles for integration of child psychiatry into the pediatric health home. Washington, DC, American Academy of Child & Adolescent Psychiatry, 2012. Available at: http://www.aacap.org/ App_Themes/ AACAP/docs/clinical_practice_center/systems_of_care/ best_principles_for_integration_of_child_psychiatry_into_the_pediatric_ health_home_2012.pdf. Accessed November 21, 2013.

McCrimmon KK: Cracking the health integration code. Health News Colorado. May 30, 2012. Available at: http://www.healthnewscolorado.org/2012/05/30/cracking-the-health-integration-code. Accessed May 26, 2014.

Meadows T, Valleley R, Haack MK, et al: Physician "costs" in providing behavioral health in primary care. Clin Pediatr 50(5):447–455, 2011

Myers KM, Palmer NB, Geyer JR: Research in child and adolescent telemental health. Child Adolesc Psychiatr Clin N Am 20:155–171, 2011

National Network of Child Psychiatry Access Programs: Existing Programs. Available at: http://nncpap.org/existing-programs.html. Accessed November 30, 2013.

Prober CG, Heath C: Lecture halls without lectures: a proposal for medical education. N Engl J Med 366(18):1657–1659, 2012

Robins DL: Screening for autism spectrum disorders in primary care settings. Autism 12:537–556, 2008

Rushton J, Bruckman D, Kelleher K: Primary care referral of children with psychosocial problems. Arch Pediatr Adolesc Med 156(6):592–598, 2002

Sanders MR, Baker S, Turner KM: A randomized controlled trial evaluating the efficacy of Triple P Online with parents of children with early onset conduct problems. Behav Res Ther 50(11):675–684, 2012

Sarvet B, Gold J, Bostic JQ, et al: Improving access to mental health care for children: the Massachusetts Child Psychiatry Access Project. Pediatrics 126:1191–1200, 2010

Schonwald A, Huntington N, Chan E, et al: Routine developmental screening implemented in urban primary care settings: more evidence of feasibility and effectiveness. Pediatrics 123:660–668, 2009

Shonkoff JP, Phillips D (eds): From Neurons to Neighborhoods: The Science of Early Childhood Development. Washington, DC, National Academy Press, 2000

Sia C, Tonniges TF, Osterhus E, et al: History of the medical home concept. Pediatrics 113:1473–1478, 2004

Szeftel R, Federico C, Hakak R, et al: Improved access to mental health evaluation for patients with developmental disabilities using telepsychiatry. J Telemed Telecare 18:317–321, 2012

Taliaferro LA, Hetler J, Edwall G, et al: Depression screening and management among adolescents in primary care: factors associated with best practice. Clin Pediatr 52:557–567, 2013

Tanner JL, Stein MT, Olson LM, et al: Reflections on well-child care practice: a national study of pediatric clinicians. Pediatrics 124:849–857, 2009

Thomas CR, Holzer CE: The continuing shortage of child and adolescent psychiatrists. J Am Acad Child Adolesc Psychiatry 45:1–9, 2006

Treo Solutions: Performance analysis: healthcare utilization of CNC-enrolled population 2007–2010. Raleigh, Community Care of North Carolina, 2012. Available at: https://www.communitycarenc.org/elements/media/related-downloads/treo-analysis-of-ccnc-performance.pdf. Accessed October 12, 2013.

Turner KM, Sanders MR: Help when it's needed first: a controlled evaluation of brief, preventive behavioral family intervention in a primary care setting. Behav Ther 37(2):131–142, 2006

Turner KM, Nicholson JM, Sanders MR: The role of practitioner self-efficacy, training, program and workplace factors on the implementation of an evidence-based parenting intervention in primary care. J Prim Prev 32(2):95–112, 2011

Unützer J: The collaborative care model: an approach for integrating physical and mental health care in Medicaid health homes. CMS Issue Brief, May 2013. Available at: http://www.medicaid.gov/State-Resource-Center/Medicaid-State-Technical-Assistance/Health-Homes-Technical-Assistance/Downloads/HH-IRC-Collaborative-5-13.pdf. Accessed October 12, 2013.

Williams J, Shore SE, Foy JM: Co-location of mental health professionals in primary care settings: three North Carolina models. Clin Pediatr 45(6):537–543, 2006

Wolraich ML, Lambert W, Doffing MA, et al: Psychometric properties of the Vanderbilt ADHD diagnostic parent rating scale in a referred population. J Pediatr Psychol 28:559–567, 2003

CHAPTER 5

Risk Management and Liability Issues in Integrated Care

Kristen Lambert, J.D., M.S.W., LICSW, FASHRM

D. Anton Bland, M.D.

In response to an increasing need for behavioral health services and improved outcomes, there is a growing shift from autonomous behavioral health and primary care practices to collaborative care practice models, which incorporate behavioral health specialists (e.g., psychiatrists, psychologists, or counselors) within primary care clinics (Wulsin et al. 2006). In addition, improving the health status of patients with serious mental illness (SMI) requires integration with primary care to be successful. The emergence of collaborative care and the potential for more reliable funding mechanisms through accountable care organizations and patient-centered medical home models are changing the way traditional psychiatry is practiced. The goal of integrated care is to provide a comprehensive treatment structure whereby primary care providers (PCPs) interact with a number of other providers, including psychiatrists, in the overall care and treatment of their patients.

This information is not intended to be and should not be used as a substitute for legal or medical advice. Rather it is intended to provide general risk management information only. Legal or medical advice should be obtained from qualified counsel to address specific facts and circumstances and to ensure compliance with applicable laws and standards.

When working as a member of a collaborative care team, it is important to clarify some malpractice liability risks as well as other general liability risks. This chapter will provide information on medical malpractice issues, including direct and vicarious liability; identify the different forms of consultation to team members; describe the duty of the psychiatrist across the spectrum of roles on the team; and make recommendations to reduce the risk of malpractice concerns. Additional emerging risks will also be identified. Bear in mind that issues regarding liability may not always be clear; however, this chapter is intended to provide a framework for some of the risk management issues to consider when working as members of collaborative care teams.

MEDICAL MALPRACTICE

Background on Medical Malpractice Cases

In most medical malpractice cases, the plaintiff (patient) or delegate (often a family member) asserts a claim for negligence against the provider. Briefly, medical malpractice is professional negligence by a doctor, nurse, or other health care worker that causes physical or emotional harm to a patient. This can result from something the provider did or otherwise failed to do.

There is a four-prong analysis that must be proven in a medical malpractice negligence case against a health care provider. Generally, in order for a plaintiff to be successful in a medical malpractice lawsuit, he or she must prove that all four elements exist. Although there may be slight variations between jurisdictions, the same basic elements apply. A litigant is either the person who files suit (the plaintiff, often the patient or next of kin in medical malpractice suits) or the person or entity being sued (the defendant, and in this context, the psychiatrist, other health care provider, corporation, clinic, etc.). If the defendant can establish that one or more of the elements do not exist, then the plaintiff will not prevail. The elements are as follows:

1. *Duty:* A duty must have been owed to the patient by the health care provider. Concerning a case specifically against a physician, a doctor-patient relationship must exist for there to be a duty (discussed in section "Doctor-Patient Relationships and Legal Duty").
2. *Breach of duty:* The health care provider who had the duty of care for the patient must have failed in his or her duty by not exercising the degree of care or medical skill that another health care professional, in the same specialty, would have used in a similar situation. Most often, expert testimony is used to demonstrate what the appropriate standard of care would be.
3. *Causation:* The breach of the health care provider's duty was causally related to the patient's injury.

4. *Damages:* The patient must have suffered an injury (physical and/or emotional).

In the event of a lawsuit, if one or more of these elements are missing, typically defense counsel will seek to have the case dismissed by the court. Some motions are available to litigants that may be "dispositive" in the sense that the litigation may be terminated without the need for a trial. In litigation where the parties agree upon the facts, the judge's function is limited to applying the law to these "undisputed" facts without the need for a jury to decide the facts. The judge can only look to see if there is a dispute. If there is no dispute, the judge may grant judgment, effectively ending the case. It will be dependent upon the court's decision, and if potentially appealed to a higher court, whether the defendant is ultimately dismissed from a lawsuit.

There are a number of other types of causes of action that can be asserted against a health care provider, which may include improper diagnosis and treatment (including failure to monitor), vicarious liability (discussed in section "Doctor-Patient Relationships and Legal Duty"), and failure to provide informed consent.

Doctor-Patient Relationships and Legal Duty

In order for there to be a legal duty, there must first be the existence of a doctor-patient relationship (Sederer et al. 1998). In other words, before a psychiatrist may be found liable for an act of medical malpractice, it is essential that a doctor-patient relationship exist (*Sterling v. Johns Hopkins Hospital* 2002).

This relationship may result from a number of situations, and it is not necessarily dependent upon the existence of a formal or "express agreement" (*Sterling v. Johns Hopkins Hospital* 2002). Generally, the psychiatrist must take some affirmative step, such as consenting to treat a patient, for the doctor-patient relationship to be established (*Sterling v. Johns Hopkins Hospital* 2002). Courts and/or juries determine whether a doctor-patient relationship occurs, and this is sometimes difficult to ascertain because it may be somewhat unclear. In the simplest form, the physician and the patient both agree to examination, diagnosis, prescribing, and/or treatment. However, a doctor-patient relationship can potentially be established even if the physician sees the patient on one occasion in consultation, which often occurs in the classic consultation-liaison service seen on inpatient medical-surgical units in hospital settings.

Courts have created factors to determine whether a physician-patient relationship exists. It is important to note that once a doctor-patient relationship is established, the doctor owes a duty to the patient to provide treatment that complies with the standard of care. This duty arises irrespective of reimbursement for services.

Factors that the courts may consider include the following:

- Existence of a relationship between the consulting physician and the facility providing care that would require the consultant to provide advice (e.g., a contract between the physician and facility for services)
- Degree to which the consultation given affected the course of treatment
- Relative ability and independence of the PCP to implement his or her own decision (*Bessenyei v. Raiti* 2003). Note that there may be variations among states in determining how the courts view a doctor-patient relationship.

Courts may also impose vicarious liability under the legal doctrine of *respondeat superior* (whose Latin translation is "let the master answer for the deeds of his servant"). Under *respondeat superior,* a supervisor can be held liable (responsible) for the acts of the staff he or she supervises. For example, a psychiatrist who agrees to supervise trainees, licensed clinicians, and nonmedical therapists, or practices within a group, setting may be held liable for the actions of others within the scope of his or her practice (Simon and Shuman 2007). In essence, while a psychiatrist may have no direct involvement with a patient, if there is a leadership role, there may be vicarious liability (*Dias v. Brigham Medical Associates, Inc.* 2002) (also see section "Supervisory Role").

CONSULTATIONS IN COLLABORATIVE CARE SETTINGS

Consultations within psychiatry, and specifically integrated care settings, occur frequently because providers collaborate about patient care, and they are considered an essential part of the collaborative care model. Thus, there may be potential for liability if a consultation is provided to another clinician or directly to the patient. Physician liability may ultimately depend upon whether the physician engaged in a formal consultation or an informal consultation (often referred to as "curbside" consultation). As indicated in the section "Doctor-Patient Relationships and Legal Duty," it may not always be easily identified. Courts and juries consider many factors when determining liability. It is important to understand that liability may attach to a physician's actions, especially when the physician is using his or her clinical expertise to advise a colleague on a recommended course of treatment.

In general, there are two main ways of providing consultations on patient care: formal and informal consultation.

Formal Consultation

Formal consultation occurs when a treating physician directly requests the written and/or verbal opinion of a consulting physician, and the consultant takes an affirmative action based on this request. The consultation could be completed through a variety of methods, including, but not limited to, face-to-face interview of the patient, telephone assessment, and televideo evaluation. This results in the creation of a physician-patient relationship and a legal duty to the patient. Following the consultation, the consultant typically documents in the patient's medical record (Sederer et al. 1998) and may prescribe medications per arrangement with the requesting physician. Finally, the psychiatrist and/or the psychiatrist's employing agency may receive a fee for services rendered in the care of the patient.

Informal ("Curbside") Consultation

Informal consultation generally occurs when a treating physician seeks the informal advice of a colleague concerning a course of treatment for a patient. In these cases, the patient's identity is rarely known to the consultant (Sederer et al. 1998); the psychiatrist does not usually perform a face-to-face interview of the patient; and the psychiatrist typically provides no written documentation within the patient's medical record. The psychiatrist may review the medical record but may not interview the patient. The psychiatrist receives no compensation for services rendered in the care of the patient, and the treating physician remains in charge of the patient's care and treatment. However, the absence of compensation or direct examination does not alleviate the psychiatrist's duty to provide care within the standard of care.

Risk Management Considerations When Providing Consultations

There are a number of published cases involving curbside consultations. Whether liability attaches is dependent upon the specific facts of a case, applicable rules, regulations, case law within the state, and the court's determination (*Mead v. Legacy Health System* 2012; Olick and Bergus 2003; *Schroeder v. Albaghdadi* 2008). There typically is a lower risk of liability in an informal consultation; however, it is not always a clear-cut issue of liability because there are a number of factors that could be involved. Even if the court ultimately decides to dismiss a psychiatrist from a case because of lack of a doctor-patient relationship (no duty to the patient), it may take several years for this to occur. Curbside consultations are an integral component of practice in the collaborative care setting, particularly when treating patients that are not improving. It is important to be aware of a state's laws on curbside consultation as well as the principles of medical ethics as they relate to a particular practice.

While psychiatrists practicing in the integrated model need to be cautious, collaboration increases knowledge between providers and may be highly beneficial in the overall care and treatment of patients. There are a few issues to consider when providing any form of consultation. First, it is important to consider the contractual relationship between the consulting psychiatrist and the agency itself. The contract may identify the role of the psychiatrist within the agency to include patient care, whether the psychiatrist is in a supervisory capacity, or whether there is any administrative function such as partner or shareholder. It is important to consider if other providers are making decisions about the clinical care of the patient and to remember the PCP requesting a consultation may not be the only provider for a particular patient. If there is an adverse outcome, the roles among providers and specified roles within the contract may be at issue. Also, consider the system for addressing patient care emergencies, including threats of violence. System policies and procedures are important because they may reduce liability risk. If practitioners know what their role is in an emergency, this may reduce the overall risk both from a patient safety standpoint and also from a liability standpoint.

Another consideration is who is responsible for various aspects of the patient's care and the coverage arrangements for each clinician in his or her absence. If a provider is unavailable or if it is off hours, it is important to have a coverage system in place. For example, if a patient has an emergency and his provider is unavailable, consider having an answering service that directs him to the emergency department or have a provider who can cross-cover. It is also important to consider if the consultant's role crosses from an informal to a formal consult. When moving from an informal to formalized consult, there may be an increase in risk of liability should an adverse issue occur. However, there may be differing views on these roles, and the outcome or whether liability attaches may be dependent upon the specific facts of the case or determination by a court.

VARYING ROLES OF THE PSYCHIATRIST

As discussed throughout this chapter, there are a variety of models for practicing psychiatry in collaborative care settings. A psychiatrist within this model will engage in what is known as "split treatment" with other providers. Exploring the role of the psychiatrist in this setting, where the collaborative care team may all engage in split treatment, requires examining the three "traditional" split treatment models. It is important to be aware of the ethical guidelines when working with other providers, including nonmedical therapists (for more information, see American Psychiatric Association 2009).

Split Treatment

Split care or split treatment occurs when several providers manage the health care of the same patient. In a traditional behavioral health setting, you may have a clinic where psychologists, social workers, and psychiatrists all see a patient for the same issues but often for different purposes. For example, a patient who has major depression may see a psychologist weekly for individual therapy, a social worker monthly for family therapy, and a psychiatrist monthly for medication management. All three providers are providing an aspect of care for the same patient concurrently. Similarly, on collaborative care teams a patient with depression may see a PCP for medical issues as well as medication management for depression and a behavioral health provider (BHP) for brief psychotherapeutic interventions as well as a consulting psychiatrist if the patient is not improving and formal consultation is requested by the other providers.

Traditional Role of the Psychiatrist in a Split Treatment Model

In a traditional split treatment context, the basic role assumed by the psychiatrist may consist of one or a combination of the following: supervisory role, collaborative role, or consultative role. All three roles will be examined, and hypothetical case scenarios for each will be provided (note that the outcome of the hypothetical cases will be dependent upon the jurisdiction and the specific facts of the case).

Supervisory Role

The first split treatment role to consider is the supervisory role. In this role, the psychiatrist is the clinical and administrative supervisor of the staff reporting to him or her. This role is typically associated with the highest liability risk of the three roles because the psychiatrist is responsible for the overall care of the patient, and all clinical decisions and actions are under the psychiatrist's direction. The psychiatrist remains ethically and medically responsible for the patient's care as long as treatment continues under his or her supervision. In the supervisory role, the psychiatrist has the ability to alter treatment and give direction to clinicians under his or her supervision.

There is a wide range of education, competence, and experience among those who treat patients with mental illness. There may be less experienced providers who have direct patient involvement and who are supervised by more experienced providers. Someone in the role of a supervisor should provide oversight consistent with standard ethical, medical, and legal responsibilities. The psychiatrist should be aware of the level of education, training, and experience of the other providers to determine the amount of supervision that may be indicated. For example, more supervision may be needed for a BHP who has 2 years of clinical experience versus one who has additional education and 15 years of experience. Furthermore, it is important to be aware if there are specific regulations in a given state on the level of supervision (e.g., frequency of chart reviews or supervisory meetings) that must be provided.

Within the integrated care model, the psychiatrist may have a supervisory role over BHPs or other psychiatrists and may also supervise nurses or other nonclinical staff who directly interact with the patient. In most collaborative care settings, it is rare for the consulting psychiatrist to supervise the PCPs, although this may change in future models of health care. Adequate communication and assessment of how much oversight is needed over another individual are essential.

Within the split treatment model, if a psychiatrist supervises another provider and there is an adverse outcome resulting in a lawsuit, courts may impose liability upon the supervisor even if the supervisor had no direct involvement with the patient. In one of the most notable cases in psychiatry regarding the duty to warn, the attorney for Tarasoff commented on how the supervisory role impacted the outcome of the case:

> It is my view that if (the supervisor of the clinic) had personally examined the patient...and made an independent decision that the patient was not dangerous to himself or his victim...that there would be no cause of action based upon foreseeability. However, (the supervisor) never saw the patient...and ignored the medical records developed by his staff. (Meyer [2002] citing the attorney for Tarasoff in the *Tarasoff v Regents of the University of California* [1976] case)

In contrast, the Vermont Supreme Court held that a physician was not liable for his physician assistant's misconduct in inappropriately prescribing medications. In its opinion, the court noted that there are 39 scenarios in which a physician can be held professionally responsible, and they do not include the misconduct of a physician assistant as set forth in the case. The court focused instead on a physician's acts, namely, actions that bear on a physician's fitness and ability to practice in the state (*In re Jon Porter M.D.* 2012). Thus, there can be significant variations between states on how courts view the supervisory role. Prior to beginning a formal supervisory relationship, consider consulting an attorney if there is any uncertainty and be aware of any statutory duties applicable within your state.

Case Example: Supervisory Role

You are a psychiatrist and also a partner in a clinic that has a collaborative care team practice. You directly supervise BHPs and meet with the team weekly to discuss cases. The team is providing treatment for a 17-year-old female patient with bipolar disorder who is prescribed lithium by the PCP. She has a number of providers involved in her care and treatment. The psychiatrist has not met the patient; however, the BHP presented the case during individual supervision with the psychiatrist and has discussed her progress during weekly team meetings. Close to the end of the business day, the BHP receives a call from the patient's mother indicating her daughter is "feeling off" and her "heart is pounding out of her chest." She has no other complaints. The BHP requests that the mother bring the patient into the clinic to be seen. The BHP goes home and does not document the discussion in the medical record. The following day, the BHP checks the computer and realizes the patient did not come into the clinic. The BHP calls the patient's mother, who reports that she has the same complaints but said that she just wanted to rest. The BHP urges her to go to the emergency department or come into the clinic because the symptoms have not resolved. The patient dies the following day. The BHP is told of this and documents the second conversation in a late entry but does not document the first conversation. An autopsy shows the patient had a myocardial infarction and a secondary finding of lithium toxicity. The family files suit against several providers at the clinic, including the psychiatrist, the PCP, and the BHP, claiming that the medication caused the cardiac event and resulting death.

Issues to Consider

- The psychiatrist had no involvement with the patient but is the administrative and clinical supervisor of the BHP.
- The psychiatrist was not involved in prescribing the lithium or monitoring the patient's blood levels.
- The psychiatrist is a partner in the practice.

Collaborative Role

The second form of split treatment is the collaborative role. Collaboration in this case is an ongoing practice where a psychiatrist works together with another practitioner in the overall care of a patient, with each provider performing direct examination and independent treatment of the patient. The collaborative role is infrequently encountered in the integrated care model but is quite commonly used in traditional models of behavioral health care, where a psychiatrist may provide medication management and a psychologist provides psychotherapy. There is mutual shared responsibility for the patient with an agreement upon the diagnosis, anticipated therapies, and risks that may derive from the patient's diagnosis and treatment. Each provider has independent and interdependent duties for ongoing risk assessment, and each provider is independently licensed. There is no supervisory relationship suggested between the providers in this form of split treatment. Instead, the clinicians collaborate in the care and treatment of the patient, and each provider has a shared responsibility to tell the other about any substantive change in the patient or his or her treatment.

When engaged in a traditional collaborative role with another clinician in the care and treatment of patients, it is important to know that the other clinician has adequate liability insurance coverage. In the event that there ever is a case resulting in catastrophic injuries (such as a death or permanent injury), ensuring that each provider has adequate professional liability coverage may help lessen the risk of exposure of personal assets should a large verdict occur.

Case Example: Collaborative Role

A patient with depression is being seen in a primary care clinic by a collaborative care team and is not improving. The PCP has tried several antidepressants, and the BHP has been utilizing behavioral activation and other brief interventions. The psychiatric consultant, Dr. Smith, is asked to do a formal evaluation, and he sets aside time the following week. The BHP discussed the patient during the weekly team meeting with Dr. Smith but did not inform him the patient had checked question #9 on the Patient Health Questionnaire depression rating scale (PHQ-9) that he or she had been feeling suicidal. Dr. Smith evaluates the patient and recommends that the PCP begin treatment with an antidepressant. The PCP starts a new antidepressant as recommended by Dr. Smith. The following week the patient attempts suicide.

Issues to Consider

- The psychiatric consultant is not the supervisor of the BHP.
- The psychiatrist did a formal consultation with the patient.
- When recommending treatment changes, the roles of the providers in the overall care of the patient should be taken into account.

Consultative Role

The third split treatment role is the consultative role (for further discussion, see section "Informal ("Curbside") Consultation"). Typically, the consultative role has the least liability risk of the three traditional split treatment roles. This is not always the case, however, because liability may depend upon a number of factors, as indicated in the section "Doctor-Patient Relationships and Legal Duty." In the consultative role, the patient's treatment will likely be directed by someone other than the psychiatrist, usually the PCP. The PCP may choose to follow the advice of the psychiatrist or not, and the psychiatrist remains outside the decision-making chain of command. In other words, the PCP continues to direct the overall care of the patient and remains in charge of decision making, not the consultant psychiatrist. This role should be made clear between the providers and, where applicable, to the patient. There is no supervisory relationship between the psychiatrist and BHP or PCP in the consultative form of split treatment.

Case Example: Consultative Role

Dr. Brown is a child and adolescent psychiatrist who works 1 day per week as a consultant in a clinic providing collaborative care in a pediatric practice. Dr. Connor, a pediatrician, was hired by the practice 4 months ago and is treating an 8-year-old child with attention-deficit/hyperactivity disorder. He has tried several medications, but the child is not responding well to treatment. Dr. Connor runs into Dr. Brown in the hall, tells him about the patient, and asks for his input for other treatment options. Dr. Brown provides advice on the case and suggests that he try another medication, and they do not discuss the case again. Dr. Connor gives the patient the medication that Dr. Brown suggested, and the patient has an adverse event that leads to the family filing suit against both Dr. Brown and Dr. Connor. Dr. Brown is not Dr. Connor's supervising physician, and he is not separately involved in the treatment of the patient. Dr. Brown does not have an administrative role at the clinic.

Issues to Consider

- Dr. Brown does not know the patient, did not perform an examination of the patient, and did not directly order the suggested medication.
- Dr. Connor had the choice to use the advice given by Dr. Brown or not.
- Dr. Brown is not Dr. Connor's supervising physician and does not have an administrative role in the clinic.

Hybrid Role of the Psychiatrist in Integrated Care Settings

On the collaborative care team, a blend of the traditional split treatment models may exist at different times depending upon where the patient is along the stepped-care continuum. The consulting psychiatrist may be in a formal supervisory role with any of the team members, most likely the BHP, and in the event of an adverse outcome, liability may attach accordingly.

To date, however, there are no known published cases of medical malpractice that have been brought against psychiatrists working on collaborative care teams (Knutson et al. 2014). However, in the event that there is a medical malpractice action, a court or jury may or may not find a consulting psychiatrist liable. There are a number of factors that courts/juries may consider in determining whether there is a relationship/duty between a psychiatrist and a patient (Bland et al. 2014).

Over the course of a patient's treatment, most of the psychiatrist's time is spent in the consultative role, with the PCP and BHP typically practicing independently in the traditional collaborative care role. The psychiatrist may enter into a collaborative split treatment role when he or she performs a formal evaluation on a patient who is not improving and additional assistance is requested by the PCP or BHP. In this function, he or she may now be performing an independent face-to-face evaluation of the patient alongside the PCP and BHP, consistent with the collaborative split treatment model, which results in entering a formal consultative role. However, even in this role, the PCP remains in charge of the overall treatment, orders all tests and medications, and ultimately decides if he or she will implement the recommendations from the consulting psychiatrist's evaluation.

In addition to engaging in the varying forms of split treatment, the psychiatrist may be involved in other activities involving patient care. In the Improving Mood—Promoting Access to Collaborative Treatment (IMPACT) model (Unützer et al. 2002), psychiatrists provide regularly scheduled caseload-based supervision with the BHPs, reviewing their registry and providing input on patients who are new to treatment or those that are not improving as expected (see Chapter 3, "Role of the Consulting Psychiatrist"). The psychiatrist makes recommendations to the BHP and PCP, who may or may not incorporate these changes into the patient's treatment plan. In some programs, the psychiatrist may provide these recommendations in writing for inclusion in the patient's medical record, although this is usually not the case. Consulting psychiatrists are often compensated for this review process as part of the contract with the primary care facility.

Case Example 1: Blended Role in Integrated Care

Dr. Right is the consultant psychiatrist in an integrated care setting. He is asked by Dr. Meyer, the PCP, to see a female patient with depression who is not improving. The BHP and PCP have been providing treatment; Dr. Meyer has been prescribing antidepressant medications and has spoken with Dr. Right on the telephone about the patient several times over the past 3 months. During this time, Dr. Meyer did not request that Dr. Right evaluate the patient, and Dr. Right did not review the patient's medical record. The BHP and Dr. Right have had regularly scheduled caseload reviews that have included discussing this patient's lack of progress. Dr. Right speaks with the PCP and BHP about the patient and decides he will see her. Following a televideo evaluation, he documents his findings in the electronic medical record (EMR) and makes a recommendation to begin treatment with a new antidepressant. He does not prescribe the medication or have any additional follow-up appointments. Dr. Meyer reviews the note and prescribes the medication recommended by the consulting psychiatrist. The patient initially responds well to the treatment change but dies 2 months later of a reaction to the medication. The family files suit.

Issues to Consider

- The psychiatrist is not the supervisor of the BHP or PCP.
- The psychiatrist did not evaluate the patient, the PCP treated the patient and did not request that the psychiatrist see the patient, and the psychiatrist did not review the medical record.
- Later in the course of treatment, the psychiatrist was asked to perform a formal evaluation.
- After the formal evaluation by the psychiatrist, the PCP relied upon his treatment recommendations.
- The psychiatrist did not prescribe the medication, and the PCP remained in charge of the overall care.

Case Example 2: Blended Role in Integrated Care

Dr. Right is a psychiatrist in an integrated care setting and meets weekly with the collaborative care team. He provides clinical supervision and reviews cases with the staff. The BHP team members are supervised by the clinic director (not the psychiatrist), who is responsible for performance reviews and other administrative tasks. This week during the team meeting, they review cases and discuss treatment options. Dr. Right does not see any of the patients discussed, does not know any identifiable patient information, and does not prescribe. He does provide recommendations to the BHPs and PCPs. Dr. Right is compensated for the caseload review. Several months later, one of the patients previously discussed commits suicide. The family files suit against the PCP, BHP, the clinic, and Dr. Right.

Issues to Consider

- Recommendations are provided to the team by the consulting psychiatrist during the caseload review.
- The BHPs report directly to a clinic director and not the psychiatrist.
- The psychiatrist receives payment for time spent doing the caseload review.
- The patients are not formally evaluated, and the psychiatrist has no personally identifiable information for any of the patients discussed.

CONTRACTUAL ISSUES

Psychiatrists should be aware of any contractual agreements in providing patient care within the institution or agency where they are employed. This is also particularly important to consider when entering into partnerships with other physicians in medical practice groups. Medical practice groups may vary in structure and organization, and therefore, it may be helpful to seek legal counsel if needed.

POLICIES AND PROCEDURES

It is advisable to have policies and procedures outlining specific roles in collaborative care settings. Policies and procedures should assist team members with guidelines pertaining to their role within the organization as well as to care and treatment of patients. It is important to remember that the development of policies and procedures may be impacted by state and federal regulations and that pursuing legal assistance may be useful.

RISK MANAGEMENT TIPS

There are a number of models and differing roles for the psychiatrist on a collaborative care team. Although not an exhaustive list, some general risk management tips include the following:

- Understand your state and federal laws and regulations pertaining to the formation of doctor-patient relationships, providing consultations, and acting in the role of a supervisor. Note that regulations and laws vary among states.
- Be clear about your involvement and the way it crosses the three split treatment categories. It is important that you know your role within this treatment model and identify when you are acting in a supervisory, collaborative, or consultative role as well as how this may change through the course of treating a patient. Your role could impact the risk of liability should an adverse outcome occur.
- Within the integrated care model, the PCP should remain in charge of the overall treatment of the patient, including any ordering of medications or additional tests. The PCP may consult a psychiatrist and is free to either follow treatment suggestions or decide on an alternate course of action. Because the PCP remains in charge of the overall care, this may reduce liability risk for the psychiatrist.
- Informal consultations are not usually documented in the medical record. However, if documentation takes place, it is important to state in writing that direct examination of the patient did not occur. A disclaimer may be incorporated within the record. When drafting disclaimer language, consult an attorney to ensure that you are adhering to state and federal laws. An example of language used by consulting psychiatric providers in the Mental Health Integration Program in Washington State (http://aims.uw.edu/resource-library/psychiatric-consultant-role-and-job-description) includes the following:

  The above treatment considerations and suggestions are based on consultations with the patient's care manager and a review of information available.... I have not personally examined the patient. All recommendations should be implemented with consideration of the patient's relevant prior history and current clinical status. Please feel free to call me with any questions about the care of this patient.

- Be cautious when an informal inquiry turns into patient diagnosis and treatment because this may change your role in providing patient care. Ensure that your role is defined: formal consultation or informal (curbside) consultation. Even if an informal consultation is provided, the psychiatrist may not necessarily be immune from being added as a defendant in a lawsuit or be prevented from being held liable should an adverse outcome occur.

• Be aware of your employment contractual obligations. Prior to signing a contract, if there are questions, it may be helpful to consult an attorney to examine contractual language concerning your role and responsibilities.

• Read the organization's policy and procedures to make sure you understand the role and expectation of the psychiatric consultant. Ensure there are clear delineations of responsibility between team members and know who is supervising whom. Make sure the policies have a documentation process regarding communication with the other team members. Minimize risk where there may be potential gaps in communication.

• Adhere to your profession's ethical guidelines.

OTHER LIABILITY ISSUES

Although this chapter mainly focuses on the liability issues in the medical malpractice realm, this section provides a cursory overview of other types of lawsuits that can be brought against a health care provider or facility within the integrated care setting. These additional liability issues are broad areas that cannot be addressed fully in this context, but a brief description is provided. As with liability issues in patient care as discussed previously, policies and procedures should be implemented in an effort to mitigate risk.

General Liability

In the integrated care setting, general liability risks may also be encountered. Although many of these additional liability risks may not be applicable to psychiatrists who act as consultants and do not operate as administrators or partners or in supervisory roles, it is important to be aware of these additional general liability issues. These may include claims of breach of contract (such as issues between partners, vendors, or property owners) or personal injuries (such as slip and falls and injuries that may occur on the property). Again, laws may vary among states; if there are questions, consultation with an attorney is advised.

Employment Liability

Employment liability matters have been increasing in recent years. This may be due to environmental factors such as the economic downturn. There are a number of claims that may potentially be brought against an employer in the employment liability context. Retaliation claims, in particular, are on the rise. Additionally, some other claims may include the following: wrongful termination, sexual harassment, age discrimination, race discrimination, and disability discrimination.

Scope of Practice

An issue that may be at the forefront of concern for psychiatrists practicing in public mental health settings involves providing general medical care for patients with chronic conditions with SMI who are dying 25 years prematurely (see volume Section II, "Primary Care in Behavioral Health Settings") because of untreated health conditions, in other words, the issue of psychiatrists providing treatment that may be considered primary care in nature. Particularly in public behavioral health settings, patients may have many medical comorbidities in addition to their psychiatric diagnoses. This can be a difficult situation for psychiatrists who refer patients for medical treatment outside the behavioral health setting, who then fail to keep the follow-up appointments in the primary or specialty medical clinics. This failure to follow through is due to many barriers and can lead to a frustrating cycle of referral with continued lack of attention to medical issues. This has led some psychiatrists to decide to seek additional training and provide limited care in the behavioral health environment (Raney 2013).

Providing medical treatment outside the scope of psychiatry may be a difficult situation for the psychiatrist. The issue becomes whether the psychiatrist has a duty to treat the patient when a medical issue arises or if it is outside the area of expertise of the psychiatrist. A consideration is whether the psychiatrist is competent to treat the patient. Competency may be gained through additional education, training, experience, and/or consultation to treat the condition. It is important to keep in mind that every case is different, and in the event of a lawsuit, outcomes may also differ depending on jurisdiction and applicable rules and regulations. A more detailed discussion of psychiatrists' responsibilities in the medical treatments of patients with SMI can be found in Chapter 7 ("The Case for Primary Care in Public Mental Health Settings").

Dixon et al. (2007) note a continuum of responsibility for the psychiatrist, and if the psychiatrist is providing treatment, then he or she is responsible for awareness of potential adverse reactions to medications and must provide monitoring and intervention when indicated. This is considered to be the highest level of responsibility. Also on the continuum is the psychiatrist's responsibility to be aware of co-occurring medical conditions that can be worsened by psychiatric medications or that can exacerbate or interfere with psychiatric conditions. They note a need to identify such medical conditions and to ensure they are addressed (Dixon et al. 2007).

Next is whether the psychiatrist has a responsibility for providing preventive monitoring, screening, and education for medical conditions that negatively impact their psychiatric patients. This is an issue that is much debated (Dixon et al. 2007). Keep in mind the American Medical Association Principles of Medical Ethics (Principle I): "A physician shall be dedicated to providing competent medical care, with compassion and respect for human dignity and rights" (American Medical Association Council on Ethical and Judicial Affairs 2012–2013). If the psychiatrist does not feel competent to provide medical care and treatment for a particular condition, consider whether additional training and consultation would be required to do so. In addition, some state boards of medicine may have online resources concerning competence.

Every case is specific and the acuity of the medical issue that the patient is experiencing is a factor. In the integrated care model, particularly those with on-site primary care clinics in the behavioral health setting, there is the advantage of collaboration with PCPs in the overall care and treatment of the patient. The American Medical Association Principles of Medical Ethics (Principle V) indicate, "A physician shall continue to study, apply, and advance scientific knowledge, maintain a commitment to medical education, make relevant information available to patients, colleagues, and the public, obtain consultation, and use the talents of other health professionals when indicated" (American Medical Association Council on Ethical and Judicial Affairs 2012–2013). Consulting or collaborating with other professionals may be indicated depending upon the circumstances.

If there is an adverse outcome, it is unclear whether a psychiatrist may be held liable for providing medical care that could be considered outside his or her scope of practice or, conversely, not seeking training to develop additional skills to provide some limited assessment and treatment if necessary. This may likely depend on the specific facts of the case and court determination (for more information on this topic and for an example of taking care of a complex patient with both SMI and chronic health conditions, see Chapter 10, "Management of Leading Risk Factors for Cardiovascular Disease"). Additional issues may arise in primary care settings where a psychiatrist trained in adult care is asked by a PCP to provide consultation for someone under the age of 18. Again, pursing additional training and consultation with child and adolescent psychiatrist colleagues, as well as following evidence-based treatment algorithms (see Chapter 4, "Child and Adolescent Psychiatry in Integrated Settings"), can help prepare the psychiatrist to fulfill the role as more of a generalist in these collaborative care settings.

EMERGING ISSUES

Privacy and Security

Health Insurance Portability and Accountability Act/Health Information Technology for Economic and Clinical Health

In general, a psychiatrist's legal obligation with respect to privacy and security of patient health information (PHI) is defined by federal and state laws and the courts. The Health Insurance Portability and Accountability Act (HIPAA) Privacy Rule is the most notable. The U.S. Department of Health and Human Services (2013) published a final rule designed to strengthen the HIPAA privacy and security rules. The final rule became effective March 26, 2013, and covered entities and business associates had until September 23, 2013, to comply with most provisions. In response to the changes, the American Psychiatric Association reviewed and summarized the final rule for its members (American Psychiatric Association 2013).

It is important to note that HIPAA allows the sharing of health care information, without a signed release of information by the patient, for "care coordination." However, there may be stricter state laws on the sharing of PHI that supersede HIPAA. Individual states may have specific regulations affording higher protection to sensitive medical records (e.g., references regarding mental health diagnosis/treatment, substance abuse, HIV, and/or sexually transmitted diseases). Some states may require an additional specific release of information by the patient or a court order to allow release to other providers.

Data Breach

Privacy and security breaches are of concern and can occur within the health care arena. Data breach is an increasing liability concern, specifically if the psychiatrist is involved with patient care and stores PHI within a computerized system or handheld device. Implementing policies and procedures and training employees in the integrated care setting on how to comply with state and federal privacy laws are necessary in order to reduce the risk of a data breach, particularly because the medical records will likely involve highly sensitive behavioral health information. In addition, it is also important to utilize hardware and software security measures. For instance, when using a laptop computer and storing patient data, it is important that the data are encrypted because unencrypted data are subject to the HIPAA "breach notification" provisions, which can be costly and increase liability exposure. For further protection, "remote wipe" software can be installed and used to erase data in the event that a computer is stolen. Again, this is not a complete analysis of privacy and security issues, but it serves rather to alert the reader that this is an emerging area of risk.

Documentation

Written Documentation

There are many principles concerning written documentation and strategies that can be implemented to reduce risk. Within the collaborative care model, a psychiatrist might not provide a formal consultation, review the patient's medical record, or know the patient's identity or PHI and might never examine the patient. However, there are times when the psychiatrist will provide a formal consultation and will document in the medical record. In the event of a lawsuit, when there is a doctor-patient relationship, lack of or incomplete documentation may often be used to support a case against the provider. Conversely, documentation can assist in the defense of a case and may be the only evidence available years later. Many states have regulations on how long medical records must be kept. They should be maintained in a manner that complies with applicable regulations, accreditation standards, professional practice standards, and legal standards. Whether a provider documents or does not document is not indicative of whether he or she will be held liable should there be an adverse outcome. Liability is dependent upon the facts of the case and the outcome decided by a court or jury.

Electronic Medical Records

If the psychiatrist documents using an EMR, there are a number of issues to consider. One issue is whether the psychiatrist has access to the same EMR as the other providers or if there are limitations. The medical record may contain sensitive information and having safeguards in place to restrict access to only staff involved in the care of the patient may be indicated. However, sharing of information is often encouraged within the collaborative care model, provided doing so is in accordance with regulatory guidelines. In addition, be aware of whether there is a backup system in case of an electronic record failure.

Within the integrated care setting, if the psychiatrist documents, it is important to know who maintains the record. If the psychiatrist is an independent contractor or an employee and does document but later leaves the practice, it is important to know who will retain control of the medical record. As with written documentation, ensure that the records are retained for the prescribed time period.

CONCLUSION

Integrated care is an evolving area of practice in psychiatry. Whether or not a doctor-patient relationship is established, and where the psychiatrist is functioning in the split treatment categories, may influence the level of legal risk in this system of care. Whether there is liability for alleged medical malpractice depends upon the specific circumstances surrounding each case and the different laws, regulations, and case law for the state where the psychiatrist is practicing. Thus, the psychiatrist should be aware of state and federal laws and regulations pertaining to his or her practice as well as aware of ethical obligations.

REFERENCES

American Medical Association Council on Ethical and Judicial Affairs: Code of Medical Ethics: Current Opinions With Annotations 2012–2013. Chicago, IL, American Medical Association, 2012–2013

American Psychiatric Association: Guidelines for Psychiatrists in Consultative, Supervisory or Collaborative Relationships With Nonphysician Clinicians. Resource Document. Arlington, VA, American Psychiatric Association, 2009

American Psychiatric Association: APA Reviews Final HIPAA Privacy Rule, January 24, 2013. Available at http://www.psychiatry.org/advocacy--newsroom/advocacy/apa-reviews-final-hipaa-privacy-rule. Accessed May 27, 2014.

Bessenyei v Raiti, 266 F. Supp. 2d 408, 411-12 (D. Md.) (2003)

Bland, DA, Lambert K, Raney, L: Resource Document on Risk Management and Liability Issues in Integrated Care. Am J Psychiatry 171:5 (suppl 1–7), May 2014.

Dias v Brigham Med. Ass., Inc., 438 Mass. 317 (2002)

Dixon LB, Adler DA, Berlant JL, et al: Psychiatrists and primary caring: what are our boundaries of responsibility? Psychiatr Serv 58(5):600–602, 2007

In re Jon Porter M.D., 2010-045 Vt. (2012)

Knutson KH, Wei MH, Straus JH, et al: Medico-legal risk associated with pediatric mental health telephone consultation programs. Adm Policy Ment Health 41(2):215–219, 2014

Mead v Legacy Health System, 352 Ore. 267, 269 (Or.) (2012)

Meyer D: Split treatment and coordinated care with multiple mental health clinicians: clinical and risk management issues. Prim Psychiatry April 1, 2002. Available at http://primarypsychiatry.com/split-treatment-and-coordinated-care-with-multiple-mental-health-clinicians-clinical-and-risk-management-issues/.

Olick R, Bergus G: Malpractice liability for informal consultations. Fam Med 35:476–481, 2003

Raney L: The evolving role of psychiatry in the era of health care reform. Psychiatr Serv 64(11):1076–1078, 2013

Schroeder v Albaghdadi, Iowa Sup. LEXIS 26 (2008)

Sederer L, Ellison J, Keys C: Guidelines for prescribing psychiatrists in consultative, collaborative, and supervisory relationships. Psychiatr Serv 49:1197–1202, 1998

Simon R, Shuman D: The doctor-patient relationship. Focus (Am Psychiatr Publ) 5:423–431, 2007

Sterling v Johns Hopkins Hosp., 145 Md. App. 161, 169 (Md. Ct. Spec. App.) (2002)

Tarasoff v Regents of the University of California, 17 Cal.3d 425 (1976)

Unützer J, Katon W, Callahan CN, et al: Collaborative-care management of late-life depression in the primary care setting: a randomized controlled trial. JAMA 288:2836–2845, 2002

U.S. Department of Health and Human Services: Modifications to the HIPAA Privacy, Security, Enforcement, and Breach Notification rules under the Health Information Technology for Economic and Clinical Health Act and the Genetic Information Nondiscrimination Act; other modifications to the HIPAA rules. Fed Regist 78(17):5565–5702, 2013

Wulsin L, Söllner W, Pincus HA: Models of integrated care. Med Clin North Am 90:647–677, 2006

CHAPTER 6

Training Psychiatrists for Integrated Care

Anna H. Ratzliff, M.D., Ph.D.

Jürgen Unützer, M.D., M.P.H., M.A.

Marcella Pascualy, M.D.

There is increasing recognition that the psychiatrist workforce is insufficient to meet the mental health needs of the U.S. population (Wang et al. 2005). Integrated care models, such as collaborative care (CC) programs in which psychiatrists and other mental health professionals work closely with primary care providers (PCPs), can effectively leverage the unique expertise of psychiatrists and help them reach larger populations in need of mental health care. There is now a strong evidence base for CC for patients with common mental disorders such as depression or anxiety (Archer et al. 2012), and systems of care are increasingly looking for psychiatrists who are able to help develop and support such evidence-based programs. To serve as a consulting psychiatrist on a primary care team, psychiatrists will need to become skillful in a set of proficiencies and develop expertise to work in new ways. These new proficiencies are defined by the core principles of effective CC: patient-centered care, evidence-based care, measurement-based treatment to target, population-based care, and accountable care (introduced and discussed in detail in Chapter 1, "Evidence Base and Core Principles").

Traditional psychiatry residency programs will typically have trained a psychiatrist to be able to perform a direct consultation in which the patient is referred by a medical specialist for a diagnostic evaluation and treatment recommendations. However, to deliver care guided by the CC principles will require the development or refinement of additional proficiencies working in integrated care that are not currently part of traditional training programs. Additional CC proficiencies and training experiences are needed to prepare psychiatrists to take essential leadership and clinical roles on integrated care teams. These include proficiency in providing indirect consultation to a population of patients, training of PCPs and supporting medical and mental health staff in basic diagnostic and management skills, and leadership in developing, implementing, and supporting effective primary care teams caring for patients with comorbid medical and mental health needs. This chapter will present a discussion of the additional core proficiencies for any consulting psychiatrist and then propose educational approaches that are needed to develop a workforce proficient to work in CC settings.

CORE COMPETENCIES

Current psychiatry residency training is guided by a set of core competencies outlined by the Accreditation Council for Graduate Medical Education (ACGME; www.acgme.org/acgmeweb/Portals/0/PDFs/CPR_Impact.pdf). The ACGME lists six broad areas in which all specialties should provide education: medical knowledge, patient care, interpersonal and communication skills, practice-based learning and improvement, professionalism, and systems-based practice (Accreditation Council for Graduate Medical Education 2013). More recently, these core competencies were further defined by the ACGME–American Board of Psychiatry and Neurology Psychiatry Milestones Project (Accreditation Council for Graduate Medical Education and American Board of Psychiatry and Neurology 2013). These core competencies and milestones are used to guide residency training. In this chapter, the framework of the ACGME core competencies and milestones are used to outline the additional proficiencies (knowledge, skills, and attitudes) for both residents and practicing psychiatrists that are needed for a career as a consulting psychiatrist on an integrated care team. A summary of the learning objectives for these new proficiencies is listed in Table 6–1. In addition to providing behavioral health care in primary care settings, there is increasing recognition of the need for psychiatrists to provide better oversight of the medical care for psychiatric patients, particularly those with serious mental illness, who are dying 25 years prematurely. This subset of new proficiencies for addressing the medical care of these patients is outlined in Table 6–2.

Medical Knowledge

Working in primary care as a consulting psychiatrist on a CC team might best be characterized as a type of consultation-liaison psychiatry or psychosomatic medicine. However, much if not most training in consultation-liaison psychiatry today occurs in inpatient medical-surgical hospitals, whereas the

TABLE 6–1. Collaborative care proficiencies for providing behavioral health care in primary care settings

ACGME competencies	Knowledge	Skills	Attitudes	Key core principles of effective collaborative care
Medical knowledge	Evidence base for CC Chronic Care Model Spectrum of integrated care models and key principles of CC Epidemiology of common mental disorders that present in primary care	Development of integrated care plans Application of rating scales Selection of appropriate brief behavioral interventions for integrated care planning	Appreciation of rationale for developing CC to achieve improvement in population health outcomes	Evidence-based care Population-based care
Patient care	Differential diagnosis of behavioral health disorders commonly observed in primary care Differential diagnosis of medical disorders commonly seen in psychiatric patients Approach to treatment-refractory psychiatric disorders, especially depression and anxiety	Direct consultation Indirect assessment in collaboration with PCPs Supervision of other providers Provision of telepsychiatry Use of patient registries to facilitate clinical care Delivery of a stepped-care approach to treatment Support for care manager in providing brief behavioral interventions and health behavior change	Understanding fast-paced, high-volume world of primary care Comfort working with uncertainty Willingness to stretch skill set to serve special populations	Patient-centered team care Evidence-based care Measurement-based treatment to target

TABLE 6–1. Collaborative care proficiencies for providing behavioral health care in primary care settings *(continued)*

ACGME competencies	Knowledge	Skills	Attitudes	Key core principles of effective collaborative care
Professionalism	Commitment to evidence-based practice Evaluation of patients in a biopsychosocial context, with sensitivity to diverse populations	Serving as a BHP role model and educator for the CC team Management of challenging clinical situations and team conflicts Provision of constructive feedback to other team members	Commitment to patient-centered care Provision of accountable care for both improving access to care and a just distribution of finite resources Appreciation of primary care culture	Patient-centered team care Evidence-based care Measurement-based treatment to target Population-based care Accountable care
Interpersonal and communication skills	Components of integrated care planning Communication modalities, including notes, telephone, televideo consultations	Brief and effective communication with PCPs and other team members Application of new communication modalities to enhance clinical care Supporting engagement of ambivalent patients	Comfort as a member and leader of an interprofessional team	Patient-centered team care Evidence-based care

TABLE 6–1. Collaborative care proficiencies for providing behavioral health care in primary care settings *(continued)*

ACGME competencies	Knowledge	Skills	Attitudes	Key core principles of effective collaborative care
Practice-based learning and improvement	Quality improvement basics How integrated care may help deliver the "triple aim"	Ability to educate primary care team members about behavioral health	Identifying themselves as the source for primary care team's knowledge of current evidence-based practice in treating behavioral health disorders	Measurement-based treatment to target Accountable care
Systems-based practice	Basic work flow and system challenges in primary care setting Knowledge of local referral patterns and resources for primary care setting	Use of quality measures as part of accountable care Ability to support team building Leadership of multidisciplinary integrated care teams in primary care or behavioral health care settings	Appreciation of roles of PCPs, other clinic providers, and staff Understanding of scope of practice, liability, and billing in the integrated care setting	Measurement-based treatment to target Population-based care Accountable care

Note. ACGME=Accreditation Council for Graduate Medical Education; BHP=behavioral health provider; CC=collaborative care; PCP=primary care provider.

TABLE 6–2. Collaborative care proficiencies for improving the health status of the population with serious mental illness in behavioral health settings

	Knowledge	Skills	Attitudes	Key principles of effective collaborative care
Primary care in behavioral health settings	Spectrum of integrated care models to provide primary care in behavioral health settings	Basic knowledge of best practices and medication management of common medical conditions leading to excess mortality	Understanding of rationale for developing programs to improve medical care of behavioral health patients Accepting responsibility for greater oversight of all health care	Patient-centered team care Evidence-based care Measurement-based treatment to target Population-based care Accountable care

majority of the demand for integrated care exists in primary care and other outpatient medical settings. The education in a general adult psychiatry residency will provide a sufficient knowledge base to be able to provide straightforward assessment and treatment recommendations for patients encountered in general medical settings, based on the focus of the current medical knowledge psychiatry milestones on developing abilities around psychopathology, clinical neuroscience, psychotherapy, somatic therapies, and psychiatric practice. However, to develop expertise as a consulting psychiatrist, additional working knowledge of the epidemiology of the typical primary care behavioral health problems, the common patient presentations encountered in primary care (Barrett et al. 1988), and how to develop appropriate differential diagnoses in primary care settings, and work as part of a team, will be necessary.

Additional medical knowledge for the consulting psychiatrist would focus on an introduction to both the rationale for developing new, population-based approaches to providing behavioral health care in primary care settings and the CC core principles. Psychiatric training usually focuses on individual patients who present or are referred for care, with an emphasis on the patient-provider dyad and the development of long-term, in-depth relationships with patients. The concept of providing behavioral health services to a population of patients (e.g., a panel or caseload of patients treated in a primary care clinic) is often a novel idea because it draws more on public health concepts than on providing care to individual patients as they choose to present for treatment. An important aspect of this introductory knowledge is the concept of the Chronic Care Model (Wagner et al. 1996), which is the foundation of many of the current models of integrated care. The Chronic Care Model identifies the essential elements of a health care system that encourage high-quality chronic disease care, including application to mental health disorders. Core elements (the community, the health system, self-management support, delivery system design, decision support, and clinical information systems) foster productive interactions between informed patients who take an active part in their care and providers with resources and expertise to provide high-quality care. Understanding of concepts such as "stepped care" (Chapter 2, "The Collaborative Care Team in Action"), in which patients are systematically tracked and treatment is intensified for patients not improving as expected, and "treatment to target" using rating scales to guide clinical decision making are important aspects of integrated care. This enables psychiatrists to support the care of defined populations of patients and may make it easier for health care organizations that employ them to be accountable to payers for care provided.

Training should also include a clear foundation of the spectrum of integrated care models, including traditional consultative care, colocated care, and systematic CC (Unützer et al. 2002, 2012). This introductory material could start with the lexicon of integrated care, a tool developed by a group of experts at the National Integration Academy Council with funding from the U.S. Agency for Health Care Research and Quality (Peek and The National Integration Academy Council 2013). This lexicon helps to define many of the overlapping concepts of integrated care. An understanding of the advantages, the challenges, and the evidence base for the various approaches to integrated care is fundamental to the ability of consulting psychiatrists to understand their roles and responsibilities.

Patient Care

A major difference between traditional residency training and the CC approach is that the consulting psychiatrist will need skills in diagnosis and treatment of common behavioral health disorders as part of a team and often for patients he or she will not directly evaluate. One of the greatest challenges for a new consulting psychiatrist will be performing these indirect or "curbside" assessments and making recommendations after a presentation by a behavioral health provider (BHP) or PCP. To be able to meet the needs of large populations of patients, the consulting psychiatrist will often be leveraging his or her skill set by providing these case reviews and diagnostic or treatment recommendations for the majority of the population (95% in the initial Improving Mood—Promoting Access to Collaborative Treatment [IMPACT] trial were managed indirectly, as mentioned in Chapter 3, "Role of the Consulting Psychiatrist") without seeing the patients in person. The ability to efficiently review medical records or hear case presentations by a PCP or BHP, identify a preliminary working diagnosis, and make initial recommendations will often feel like functioning as a "backseat driver" and requires patient care skills in assessing the information available, knowing what else to ask, and developing an integrated plan from this information. There are also new proficiencies that must be learned, including when and how to "step up" care to a direct assessment either in person or using a telepsychiatry approach if patient treatment goals are not reached. The ability to perform indirect assessments and step up care, which are fundamental to the CC principles of population-based care and measurement-based treatment to target, is most consistent with achieving a level 4 or 5 on the current patient care psychiatry milestones. This requires the ability to synthesize information into a concise formulation, choose the appropriate level of care, and teach or support another team member in the implementation of the integrated care plan.

A key element in this "indirect process" is the use of registries to facilitate patient care. This involves using an electronic database to track key clinical and quality-of-care outcomes of a specific population of patients in order to determine which patients need additional consultation, in-person evaluation, treatment changes or intensification, or referral to additional specialty behavioral health services. Knowledge of registries and practice with using them to guide care of a population will be an important skill to master to be able to meet the principles of population-based care and measurement-based treatment to target.

Another new patient care proficiency is to become familiar with the wide variety of chief complaints that are not typical of patients presenting in mental health clinics, such as unexplained and persistent somatic complaints, and often must be differentiated from physical health problems. Increasingly, primary care settings are using brief, validated screening instruments such as the nine-item Patient Health Questionnaire depression rating scale (PHQ-9; Kroenke et al. 2001) to identify patients with common mental health disorders. Familiarity with the use of such screening tools to aid in case finding, diagnosis, and monitoring of treatment for a variety of common mental disorders is a key skill for an integrated care team and the consulting psychiatrist (other common screeners are listed in Chapter 2). In addition to familiarity with the most common behavioral health disorders observed in primary care settings, the consulting psychiatrist will need to help the primary care team differentiate mental health disorders from other common presentations such as distress, demoralization (Griffith and Gaby 2005), or maladaptive health behaviors that complicate the treatment of common medical problems. This often requires the consulting psychiatrist to educate the BHP on a systematic approach to the differential diagnosis and diagnostic criteria. Important considerations will be assessing for important rule-out diagnoses (e.g., bipolar disorder in depressed patients) and medical illness that can mimic psychiatric illness (e.g., patients with hypothyroidism can present as depressed or patients with hyperthyroidism can present with anxiety) or effects of medications (such as depression related to initiation of interferon treatment for hepatitis C).

Developing an appreciation of the fast-paced, high-volume world of the primary care team is necessary to be able to provide realistic guidance for medical decision making. For example, sessions are often shorter in primary care settings, so limiting the assessment to critical questions that need to be answered before a treatment is initiated is a common primary care approach. This is often quite different from the typical 60- to 90-minute initial psychiatric intake appointment and requires development of comfort with an iterative process of assessment and recommendations (Figure 6–1) in which a complete diagnostic formulation and treatment plan emerges only after a series of brief successive contacts with the PCP and a supporting BHP and consultation with the psychiatrist. Key attitudes of comfort with uncertainty and flexibility must be developed in the consulting psychiatrist to be able to deliver care using this approach. One of the important principles that must be explored by the consulting psychiatrist is balancing the tension between the need for complete information and the risk of not acting or making a recommendation. In a primary care setting, the consulting psychiatrist will need to become comfortable with "ruling out" high-risk conditions early on and then trusting the team to initiate a preliminary treatment plan even in the absence of a "perfect" diagnosis. As long as there is close and systematic follow-up by the team, a more complete diagnostic picture often emerges over time, and appropriate adjustments can be made with recommendations from the consulting psychiatrist.

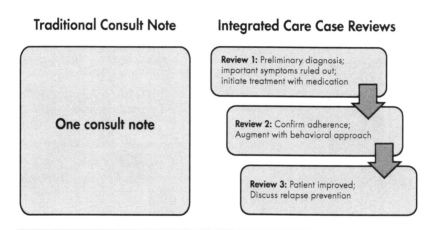

FIGURE 6–1.   Illustration of how the integrated care case review approach is an iterative process, giving several opportunities to impact treatment, compared with a single comprehensive evaluation.

Source.   Copyright 2013 University of Washington. Used with permission.

An extension of the current patient care milestones is the proficiency to provide both somatic and psychotherapeutic treatment for a wide spectrum of behavioral health conditions in primary care settings. Continuing to learn about current advances is critical to be able to achieve the CC principle of ensuring the whole team is providing evidence-based care. Because the majority of common mental health conditions such as depression and anxiety can be treated by a PCP and supporting behavioral health staff such as a BHP in primary care, the consulting psychiatrist will often be asked to focus on and support treatment for patients with refractory mental health disorders, such as depression and anxiety, that are not responding to initial medication treatment or psychotherapy. Developing a systematic approach to treating refractory depression and anxiety and familiarity with current evidence-based best practices for treating common behavioral health disorders are essential to perform this function. Helping a primary care team assess for common causes of nonresponse to medication interventions (such as a misdiagnosis, inadequate doses of medication, need for a different medication, difficulty obtaining medication, interference because of substance use, and difficulty with medication adherence) and recommending evidence-based psychotherapy or other behavioral interventions can be vital to treating behavioral health disorders to remission.

The consulting psychiatrist also needs skills in supporting the delivery of brief behavioral interventions that have been proven effective in primary care settings, for example, motivational interviewing, behavioral activation, problem-solving therapy, and health behavior change intervention such as smoking cessation. The role for the consulting psychiatrist will often be to support another provider to deliver such evidence-based interventions, with a particular focus on teaching the fundamentals of these skills, referral to community resources for such behavioral interventions, or problem solving if a patient is not responding to initial treatment. The primary care team often looks to the consulting psychiatrist as a health behavior expert, and the consulting psychiatrist must develop a breadth of brief behavioral intervention skills that go beyond the management of common psychiatric disorders and include the management of maladaptive health behaviors. Ability to perform this role as teacher and supervisor is consistent with achieving a level 4 or 5 on the current patient care psychiatry milestones.

An ability to make recommendations to a variety of populations will often challenge consulting psychiatrists to "stretch their skill set." Consulting psychiatrists are often asked by their colleagues in primary care to make recommendations for populations that they may have little experience with, such as pregnant or geriatric patients, or in areas that have traditionally been considered subspecialties, such as addictions, chronic pain, or child and adolescent psychiatry (see Chapter 4, "Child and Adolescent Psychiatry in Integrated Settings"). Requests for recommendations for such populations will be especially common in low-resource settings such as safety net clinics or rural settings.

Professionalism

Because the psychiatrist is a clinical leader and ambassador for behavioral health care, it is especially important that the consulting psychiatrist be able to demonstrate professionalism as defined in the professionalism milestones (demonstrating compassion, integrity, respect for others, and accountability to self, patients, colleagues, and the profession) and the 10 professional responsibilities associated with professionalism in medicine as outlined by the

Charter on Medical Professionalism established by leaders in the American Board of Internal Medicine Foundation, the American College of Physicians–American Society of Internal Medicine Foundation, and the European Federation of Internal Medicine (American Board of Internal Medicine Foundation et al. 2002). Developing a commitment to several core aspects of professionalism is particularly important to the consulting psychiatrist, including committing to lifelong learning, understanding the roles and responsibilities of the team, giving functional feedback, and creating an environment of respect. In many ways, professionalism is fundamental to achieving all of the CC principles because the psychiatric consultant often represents the behavioral health role model for the entire primary care team.

A consulting psychiatrist needs to make a commitment to lifelong learning and recognize the importance of staying up to date with advances in medical knowledge and applicable research findings that will inform and improve patient care. This is particularly important in the emerging field of integrated care, where new studies, models, and techniques are being published on a frequent basis. This needs to be a core commitment because the consulting psychiatrist is responsible for determining best practices for behavioral health and helping other team members implement such practices as defined by the CC principle of evidence-based care. An example of this commitment to learning is the responsibility of the consulting psychiatrist to ensure that the BHPs are making good judgments based on accurate assessments and a sound knowledge base. Appropriate use of technology to facilitate the acquisition and sharing of knowledge with other team members will further streamline delivery of care, ensuring that everyone is working effectively and in tandem.

Another key to the success of the integrated care team is to define and understand the precise roles and responsibilities of each team member so that expectations can be met, communication and "'handoffs" are safe and effective, and appropriate feedback is given if adjustments are necessary to help members perform competently. The integrated team works collaboratively, blending multiple professional cultures to create a new one that works synergistically. This "new professional culture" needs to be viewed as a dynamic process fueled by the knowledge that the common goal of providing excellent patient care can be achieved only by learning to work effectively together as a team.

Feedback is necessary and should be viewed as an expected element in the developmental process of building a highly functional team. Members should be aware of the importance of the feedback process beforehand and view it as a building block in the continuous improvement process of achieving good working relations and improved patient care outcomes. The consulting psychiatrist may need to acquire new skills in how to provide feedback in a nonjudgmental way and should also be receptive to feedback about his or her own effectiveness as a team member in this process. The consulting psychiatrist needs to view providing feedback as a required and sometimes difficult skill that necessitates focus and a thoughtful and deliberate approach. The goal is to foster a safe and nurturing environment where exchange of information has high fidelity and where feedback is welcomed and expected and ultimately viewed as an opportunity to learn, a vital step in professional improvement. The overarching goal of promoting constructive feedback is to optimize team functioning, to safeguard patient welfare, and to achieve better patient treatment outcomes consistent with the CC principle of accountable care.

Professionalism in medicine has been associated with traits such as honesty, accountability, altruism, service, and commitment to excellence (Mitchell et al. 2012). The consulting psychiatrist must develop a professional attitude of genuine respect for others and their role on the integrated care team for effective team-based care to occur. With regard to the integrated care team, it is important to follow through with commitments, to be available when needed, and to not make inappropriate demands that are beyond the scope of team members' skills, job description, or duty hours. A consulting psychiatrist must learn to be aware of his or her own stress and to manage it in a way that does not impact the treatment team. Focusing on being courteous and remembering to express appreciation of the work and dedication and commitment of the team demonstrate humility and reduce potential hierarchical tension. Recognizing and verbalizing that the team cannot function without each and every member is validating and reminds others that the work of the team is a shared effort. Functioning at this level would typically be consistent with level 5 professionalism psychiatry milestones.

Interpersonal and Communication Skills

Effective interpersonal skills are at the core of becoming a successful consulting psychiatrist because they are essential to providing clear communication, team building, forming collegial alliances, promoting mutual respect, providing education when appropriate, and sharing in the care of the patient. The interpersonal and communication psychiatry milestones focus on relationship development, conflict management, and information sharing, which are particularly relevant to the role of consulting psychiatrist on a CC team. The different modalities a team may use to communicate, as well as strategies to optimize communication, are core content for training a consulting psychiatrist. Although most psychiatrists will be familiar with situations in which communication exchange occurs face-to-face, much of the communication used by an integrated care team occurs via telephone, televideo, or electronic forms such as e-mail, text, and electronic medical records. New proficiencies in using these technologies appropriately will include both learning how to communicate effectively, such as awareness of tone of voice, as well as limitations of these forms of communication, for example, when to use the phone or e-mail. A consulting psychiatrist must also carefully consider the structure for communication. Scheduling regular consultation, starting and ending meetings in a timely fashion, and utilizing organizational strategies will help the team with time management and efficiency. Strong written communication is another key skill, because clear and concise recommendations are more likely to ensure that treatment plans are accurate and viable.

Approaches to communicating, in the face of differing opinions, warrant a particularly important focus. Adjusting treatment plans takes tact and practice, particularly when the PCP or BHP may have just seen the patient and is proposing a treatment plan that is different from the plan proposed by the consulting psychiatrist. In this instance, learning to skillfully explain your reasoning is crucial to improve understanding, foster learning, maintain a good working relationship, and minimize unnecessary conflict. If treatment differences continue, training around when and how to step up care is a vital skill set. Like professionalism, strong interpersonal skills support all of the CC principles, and an effective consulting psychiatrist would be functioning at a level 4 or 5 on the interpersonal skills psychiatry milestones.

Practice-Based Learning and Improvement

The goals of practice-based learning and improvement are consistent with the need for the consulting psychiatrist to commit to lifelong learning and quality improvement as embodied by the CC principles population-based care, measurement-based treatment to target, evidence-based care, and accountable care. Although skills in self-evaluation and reflection are core features for psychiatric training, specific knowledge of how to lead quality improvement efforts may be new to some consulting psychiatrists. A working knowledge of and skills to engage in habitual quality improvement efforts, such as plan-so-study-act cycles (Varkey et al. 2007), at the individual and system level are needed. The ability to identify systems challenges to patient improvement can be the key to supporting a team in achieving excellent treatment outcomes. Integrated care has been proven to be able to deliver the "triple aim" of improved patient outcomes, improved patient satisfaction, and reduced costs. However, only through routine practice of outcomes tracking and quality improvement will individual teams be able to achieve this standard not only for individual patients but for the entire population of patients they care for.

Another important feature of practice-based learning is the commitment to providing the highest standards of evidence-based medical practice and to educating other providers. Many primary care teams will come to rely on the consulting psychiatrist to provide education about mental health diagnoses and treatments, differential diagnosis, pharmacological management of common psychiatric disorders, basic preventive care, and management of chronic medical disorders, including medical management and supporting lifestyle change. It will be important for the consulting psychiatrist to be able to provide best practice protocols on medication and psychotherapeutic treatments. Being able to deliver care at this level would likely require a consulting psychiatrist to perform at a level 4 or 5 on practice-based learning and improvement psychiatry milestones.

Systems-Based Practice

Because more psychiatrists are working in organized settings than in private practice, psychiatrists will likely have been introduced to the notion of systems of care as a resident. The importance of the ability to function as part of an integrated care team or consult to nonpsychiatric medical providers is the focus of the systems-based practice (SBP4) psychiatry milestone. However, the concepts of systems-based care can be challenging to understand, and recent work has been done to help define a model of systems-based practice for psychiatry (Ranz et al. 2012). In the proposed model, there are four key roles for the psychiatrist that must be considered: team member, information integrator, resource manager, and patient care advocate. The consulting psychiatrist will need to become competent in all these roles to fulfill the CC principles and to provide a more systematic approach to delivery of mental health services, facilitating the delivery of this care and improving the behavioral health of a designated population of patients.

As a team member, the consulting psychiatrist will need to understand the primary care setting and support a mental health work flow within that setting. Early in a new program, the role of the consulting psychiatrist may be to help facilitate building a strong team. Later, this role may change to supporting the team, assessing for burnout, and addressing systems issues to continue to have strong teamwork.

To perform as an information integrator and patient care advocate, the consulting psychiatrist will need a clear understanding of the tasks that must be completed by this team to provide behavioral health care in a primary care setting and how each team member will work to support the goal of improved patient outcomes. Often key quality measures, for example, the number of assessments, number of follow-ups, and percentage of patients improved, are used to assess the team's efficacy in delivering care. This concept is closely related to practice-based learning and improvement, although the focus is on improving the system rather than improving an individual patient's care. The consulting psychiatrist is ideally positioned to support systems-level evaluation because the caseload review function allows a population-level perspective. This role will be especially important to achieving the CC principle of accountability for care.

The consulting psychiatrist, as a resource manager, may help with a variety of common issues that arise when providing behavioral health care to populations of patients. Knowledge of the local referral patterns and community resources can often help the team in finding appropriate dispositions for patients for whom care needs are in excess of the capabilities of the primary care setting. Skills in developing protocols for common concerns such as suicidality help the consulting psychiatrist support the important systems-based practice goal of patient safety. Last, the complexity of scope of practice, liability risk, and mechanism for payment for providing a range of consultation services are common topics that need to be addressed by any new consulting psychiatrist.

EDUCATIONAL APPROACHES

General Residency Training

Although the focus of this chapter is training a workforce to be prepared to function as consulting psychiatrists, there are several aspects of integrated care models that may make integrated care an ideal venue to teach the psychiatry core competencies and milestones. Medical knowledge and patient care training opportunities in CC include the opportunity to work with an attending physician and to demonstrate the ability to manage outpatient treatment and provide supervision and support of a BHP reviewing multiple cases. This experience provides an opportunity both to practice psychiatry skills and apply knowledge to more patients in a condensed time and to potentially achieve level 4 or 5 for these psychiatry milestones, which typically require supervising and teaching other providers.

Participating on an interprofessional CC team will develop competencies in interpersonal and communication skills, practice-based learning and improvement, and systems-based practice, which can be difficult to teach and observe at more traditional outpatient psychiatry training sites. There are evidence-informed guidelines for creating this type of training experience, including outlined potential goals and objectives and teaching methods for integrated care (Yudkowsky and Schwartz 2000) and the description of shared mental health care efforts at McMaster University in Hamilton, Ontario

(Kates 2000). The opportunity to gain additional training in nonpsychiatric medicine (Wright 2009) may be another potential benefit of training in CC that would benefit all psychiatric residents.

At a minimum, residents should have didactic presentations about the evidence base and spectrum of approaches to integrated care. However, some research suggests that observing an attending physician at work may provide a better learning experience (De Groot et al. 2000). For example, the University of California at Davis program trains all residents in integrated care using faculty who are trained in family medicine/psychiatry or internal medicine/ psychiatry to provide psychiatric consultation and outpatient medicine in primary care and public psychiatry settings (Onate et al. 2008). Additionally, creating residency training opportunities in CC may be the optimal way to achieve level 4 and 5 competencies in the psychiatry milestones in systems-based practice, especially SBP4: consultation to nonpsychiatric medical providers and nonmedical systems. For example, Mount Sinai School of Medicine created a yearlong elective rotation to teach residents how to deliver primary care–based psychiatric services (Cerimele et al. 2013). In this rotation, residents provided direct patient care in a primary care setting, supervised a care manager, and participated in team meetings. Learning objectives included skills in consultation, techniques in teamwork, and measurement-based practice and leadership, consistent with the proficiencies needed to achieve the CC principles and learn systems-based practice.

Advanced Residency Training in Integrated Care

In addition to exposing all residents to the basic elements of practicing integrated care, residency programs are projected to experience an increasing demand to offer specialized training and clinical experiences for residents interested in pursuing careers in this area of expertise. Elective rotations in integrated care would ideally use the outline of skills, attitudes, and knowledge presented in the section "General Residency Training" to guide their educational goals and objectives. Training programs that already have established integrated care programs have begun to provide a variety of elective opportunities, which can be used as models for programs planning to establish integrated care training (Cowley et al. 2014). Some of these programs focus on colocated care opportunities, such as Cambridge Health Alliance, where residents spend rotation time working in a primary care setting. The advantage of this type of program is that residents can begin to develop a sense of the primary care world in a format that is fairly easy to establish. A subspecialty program at the Johns Hopkins Division of Child and Adolescent Psychiatry in Baltimore, Maryland, paired pediatrics and child psychiatry to allow child psychiatry fellows to be colocated and work closely with pediatric residents to learn skills to become consultant psychiatrists in an urban general pediatrics clinic (Cowley et al. 2014). Other programs, such as the Portland VA Medical Center Psychiatry Primary Medical Care Program, were designed to teach residents to provide both psychiatric and medical care to patients in an elective primary care psychiatry rotation (Dobscha et al. 2005). Programs with more fully developed CC programs, such as the University of Washington Mental Health Integration Program, offer specialized rotations to train residents to function as consulting psychiatrists in a statewide program (Cowley et al. 2014).

University of Washington Collaborative Care Rotation

This 6-month, half-day clinical rotation introduces a senior resident to the role of the consulting psychiatrist on a CC team. In this model, the team consists of a patient, a care manager embedded in a primary care setting (usually a medical social worker or other BHP), the PCP (both the source of referrals and the prescriber of any medications), and a consulting psychiatrist (providing weekly caseload supervision and individual case reviews of four to six patients weekly). During this clinical rotation, each week the resident works directly with an attending consulting psychiatrist to participate in a 1- to 2-hour consultation with a care manager (using the telephone), receives 1 to 2 hours of supervision with the attending physician, and may participate in interdisciplinary care team meetings. The supervision time includes reviewing assigned readings, discussion of a 20- to 30-minute didactic module, and the opportunity to discuss consultation observations and experiences. Close supervision is important in this rotation because for many residents, this may be their first experience with indirect evaluation of patients. Working closely with a practicing consultant psychiatrist allows the resident the opportunity to gradually assume the role of the primary consultant to a care team over the course of the rotation. To support this clinic work, residents are taught from a set of six mini-modules (slide sets and readings that can be reviewed in ~20 minutes) to cover the fundamentals necessary to assume the role of a consulting psychiatrist. After these introductory modules have been reviewed, the didactic portion of the supervision hour is devoted to individualized topics relevant to reviewed patient cases. This curriculum trains a psychiatrist to function in many roles at the interface of primary care and behavioral health. The curriculum for this rotation is available at aims.uw.edu.

Educational strategies for all the resident training experiences will need to consider the unique primary care settings available within the training programs to maximize learning. In general, psychiatry residents benefit from learning experiences in which they are both directly supervised and in which they have the opportunity to learn from observing attending psychiatrists at work (De Groot et al. 2000). One of the important barriers to consider is that many residency programs may not have established integrated care programs or have supervising attending psychiatrists who are trained sufficiently to teach residents in this area. Even when there is the opportunity and support to develop integrated approaches, there are other common barriers, such as space and attending time to provide supervision, which must be considered when an integrated care rotation is designed (Dobscha and Ganzini 2001). To meet this challenge, programs may need to invest in developing this expertise among faculty psychiatrists. Other factors to consider are the need for specific preparation for working in primary care settings, frequent misunderstandings of the psychiatry resident's role, and challenges with communication with multiple clinic providers encountered in primary care settings (Cowley et al. 2000). In order to meet these challenges, designing specific didactic experiences to address the practical details of the medical knowledge and patient care sections of the psychiatry milestones as encountered in integrated care, especially the culture of primary care settings and communication strategies for working in these settings, would make these rotations most successful.

Psychiatry Resident's Experience of Training in Integrated Care

This rotation was a great opportunity to see a different kind of service model. Thinking about how to "see" patients in this fashion and balancing this with an obligation to keep track of a larger patient panel were unique challenges that I hadn't faced before. This model also provides exposure to a large volume of patients, which is nice for experience's sake. I was surprised at how sick many of these patients were. In many ways, they were more ill than those seen in mental health clinics, I suspect because to reach a traditional psychiatric clinic, patients have to be sufficiently functional to keep a referral appointment. Then, what was impressive was that severe pathology can be managed through CC. Learning a CC approach was helpful in giving me a better sense of how primary care clinics run and, thus, what mental health care looks like for most patients. Learning this model really helped me better understand who can be managed successfully in primary care, who needs referral, and how to best utilize a range of available providers.

Fourth-year resident, Mental Health Integration Program rotation
University of Washington

In the future, residency programs could consider offering a new type of psychiatric residency track in which the majority of medical and psychiatric training would be conducted in integrated outpatient sites. For example, residents could complete their core medicine rotations in the outpatient setting to gain insight into the world of primary care, rotate through traditional inpatient and outpatient psychiatry, spend their required consultation-liaison training time in the primary care setting instead of on inpatient units, and then spend the majority of elective time in various integrated care settings.

Fellowship Opportunities in Collaborative Care

For trainees who wish to pursue advanced training opportunities, there are several fellowship tracks that could provide relevant specialized training. Integrated care has consultation-liaison psychiatry at its roots, and a fellowship in psychosomatics could be an ideal training program, especially if there were rotation opportunities to learn integrated care. Advanced training could expose the fellow to other aspects of consultative psychiatry, such as proactive approaches for high utilizers of health care, delirium prevention, and integrated case management for complex inpatients who return to primary care settings on discharge. Other fellowships oriented toward special populations, such as child psychiatry (see Chapter 4, "Child and Adolescent Psychiatry in Integrated Settings"), addictions, and geriatrics, could provide expertise that would be invaluable in the role as a consulting psychiatrist, as there is even more need for psychiatric support for these populations in primary care settings. For trainees interested in policy or research, training in public psychiatry or a research fellowship such as the health services or primary care psychiatry programs (e.g., the Psychiatry in Primary Care Fellowship at the University of Washington, www.uwpsychiatry.org/education/primary.html) may be an ideal training prospect.

PSYCHIATRISTS IN PRACTICE

Because there is increasing demand for integrated care, practicing psychiatrists will need training opportunities to gain the knowledge, skills, and attitudes required to transition to practice as a consulting psychiatrist. The most common scenario is likely to be a psychiatrist who spends part of his or her time working with primary care practices and the rest in more traditional roles. For these psychiatrists, training opportunities offered at professional meetings provide an excellent way to not only learn about these models but also network with other psychiatrists in the field and the team of experts doing the presentations. For example, a course called The Integration of Primary Care and Behavioral Health: Practical Skills for the Consulting Psychiatrist is offered at the American Psychiatric Association and the Academy of Psychosomatic Medicine meetings and other professional meetings several times annually and represents an opportunity to get an overview of this emerging career (slides from previous presentations are available on the Advancing Integrated Mental Health Solutions (AIMS) Web site at uwaims.org/training-consulting_psychiatrists.html). There are also opportunities to access training materials and webinars through national organizations such as the Substance Abuse and Mental Health Services Administration–Health Resources and Services Administration Center for Integrated Health Solutions (www.integration.samhsa.gov/workforce/training). The AIMS Center at the University of Washington has additional training and resource materials for consulting psychiatrists (aims.uw.edu).

TRAINING IN TEAMS

One of the most unique aspects of training as a consulting psychiatrist is the opportunity to gain experience participating as a member of a CC team. Psychiatrists may have an important role to champion interprofessional education as liaisons between medical and behavioral health team members (Shaw and Blue 2012), and the consulting psychiatrist may have even more opportunity to fill this important role. There are some published models of interprofessional education that can be used to support efforts to build strong integrated care teams to deliver mental health. For example, Memorial University in St. John's, Newfoundland, Canada, used a Collaborative Mental Health Practice Interprofessional Education Module, which included medical, nursing, and allied health staff and was demonstrated to be feasible and well received by trainees (Curran et al. 2012). The use of standardized patients enhanced satisfaction with the module, suggesting that incorporating such case-based teaching approaches may be useful in teaching interprofessional integrated care. Other approaches, such as Team Strategies to Enhance Performance and Patient Safety (STEPPS) training to improve patient safety through enhanced communication and other teamwork skills, may be helpful to training as an integrated care team (Clancy and Tornberg 2007). This model uses a multifaceted, multimedia instructional model including classroom teaching, PowerPoint presentations, videos, role-playing, case studies, coaching exercises, and a pocket guide to teach teamwork. These interprofessional approaches will be especially important to develop core competencies: interpersonal and communication skills, practice-based learning and improvement, and systems-based practice (for more on team development, see Chapter 2).

MEDICAL CARE IN BEHAVIORAL HEALTH SETTINGS

Although the majority of the evidence base for integrated care is focused on providing behavioral health care in primary care settings, there is a growing interest and evidence base for psychiatrists to support integration of primary care into behavioral health settings (Scharf et al. 2013). Finding system-based approaches to meet the needs of mental health patients is necessary to try to target the increased mortality seen in patients with serious mental illness (Druss et al. 2011). Many of the core proficiencies, including the core principles of CC discussed above, will be important for the psychiatrist supporting primary care in behavioral health settings; however, there are several unique aspects to providing primary care in these settings that require specialized education (Raney 2013). The setting for most of these programs will be with a PCP who is located in or near a community mental health setting. Care provided in a community mental health setting may be quite different than in a typical primary care setting, and the psychiatrist in this type of program will need to be familiar with the developing models of integrated care work flows that can be provided in behavioral health settings (see the section "Core Competencies"). In these models, there is increasing demand to have psychiatrists assume some oversight of the patients' total health care in addition to their psychiatric care. An overview of the medical care for the most common conditions leading to increased cardiovascular risk is presented in Chapter 10 ("Management of Leading Risk Factors for Cardiovascular Disease"). There may be unique challenges to provide training for this type of work; one training program has shown that although cross-training in primary care settings affects the resident's preparedness and career choice, it appeared insufficient to influence practice behaviors related to delivering general medical care (Dobscha et al. 2005). Models such as TEAMcare (Katon et al. 2010) and medical home models made available by the Patient Protection and Affordable Care Act (see Chapter 9, "Behavioral Health Homes") may provide a framework to structure care delivery where the psychiatrist works together with a PCP as a consultant for the care of patients. Having both a PCP attending and a psychiatry attending may be especially important, as preliminary findings from the Veterans Health Administration system note that an attending psychiatrist practicing alone may not be comfortable providing supervision for primary care services (Rohrbaugh et al. 2009). Finding opportunities to provide this type of integrated care will be especially relevant to workforce development so that psychiatrists understand their role when primary care services are offered in their facility or when patients are referred for primary care treatment. With this training, psychiatrists may play an important role in orienting and supporting primary care staff by helping to bridge the culture gap between behavioral health and primary care settings, and this role of helping with primary care staff may help to overcome the barrier of difficulty recruiting and retaining primary care staff as seen in the Primary and Behavioral Health Care Integration grantee programs (Chapter 8, "Providing Primary Care in Behavioral Health Settings") (Scharf et al. 2013).

FUTURE DIRECTIONS

Health care reform creates increasing pressure for our health care system to serve large populations of patients more effectively while limiting the overall cost of health care. For the millions of patients with behavioral health disorders who do not receive care from psychiatrists or other mental health specialists, evidence-based CC programs can help psychiatrists address these needs not only nationally but globally. Training a workforce to support such evidence-based team care is becoming an important educational challenge. In addition to working and leveraging the psychiatrists' unique skills more efficiently, working as part of an effective team can create highly rewarding roles for psychiatrists who appreciate their ability to contribute to the larger health care system and experience the success of helping greater numbers of patients. Effectively sharing the joy of this work may also become an important way for psychiatry to help attract some of the best and brightest medical students to our profession. Trainees who are interested in psychiatry but are concerned about losing touch with the rest of medicine may be attracted by a rotation in which a well-trained psychiatrist practices alongside other medical colleagues in a primary care setting, observing the consulting psychiatrist in a role where he or she is clearly valued and respected for his or her behavioral health expertise and contributions to the overall health care of patients.

CONCLUSION

This chapter presents a review of the new proficiencies in CC principles and training methods needed to develop a workforce prepared to deliver integrated care. In addition to these proficiencies, a successful consulting psychiatric provider will need to have developed new attitudes about what it means to work as a psychiatrist. Personal attributes of flexibility, creativity, adaptability, and tolerance will be needed in the dynamic primary care environment. The ability to work well in teams as both an educator and consultant is critical for this role because the majority of the work is with PCPs and other behavioral health professionals such as clinical social workers, psychologists, and licensed counselors. For psychiatrists who have these characteristics, the reward of practicing on a CC team is immense. Consulting psychiatrists enjoy the pace and variety of the work, the mix of direct and indirect patient contact, the caseload-based supervision and consultation that allows them to reach a larger population, training other health professionals, and the deep sense of satisfaction from working as part of a team, accountable for the care they are providing for patients.

REFERENCES

Accreditation Council for Graduate Medical Education: ACGME common program requirements. July 1, 2013. Chicago, IL, Accreditation Council for Graduate Medical Education, 2013. Available at: http://www.acgme.org/acgmeweb/Portals/0/PFAssets/ProgramRequirements/CPRs2013.pdf. Accessed December 21, 2013.

Accreditation Council for Graduate Medical Education, American Board of Psychiatry and Neurology: The Psychiatry Milestone Project, November 2013. Chicago, IL, Accreditation Council for Graduate Medical Education, 2013. Available at: https://www.acgme.org/acgmeweb/Portals/0/PDFs/Milestones/PsychiatryMilestones.pdf. Accessed January 12, 2013.

American Board of Internal Medicine Foundation, American College of Physicians–American Society of Internal Medicine Foundation, European Federation of Internal Medicine: Medical professionalism in the new millennium: a physician charter. Ann Intern Med 136(3):243–246, 2002

Archer J, Bower P, Gilbody S, et al: Collaborative care for depression and anxiety problems. Cochrane Database of Systematic Reviews 2012, Issue 10. Art. No.: CD006525. DOI: 10.1002/14651858.CD006525.pub2.

Barrett JE, Barrett JA, Oxman TE, et al: The prevalence of psychiatric disorders in a primary care practice. Arch Gen Psychiatry 45(12):1100–1106, 1988

Cerimele JM, Popeo DM, Rieder RO: A resident rotation in collaborative care: learning to deliver primary care–based psychiatric services. Acad Psychiatry 37:63–64, 2013

Clancy CM, Tornberg DN: TeamSTEPPS: assuring optimal teamwork in clinical settings. Am J Med Qual 22(3):214–217, 2007

Cowley DS, Katon W, Veith RC: Training psychiatry residents as consultants in primary care settings. Acad Psychiatry 24(3):124–132, 2000

Cowley DS, Dunaway K, Forstein M, et al: Teaching psychiatry residents to work at the interface of mental health and primary care. Acad Psychiatry April 15, 2014 [Epub ahead of print]

Curran V, Heath O, Adey T, et al: An approach to integrating interprofessional education in collaborative mental health care. Acad Psychiatry 36(2):91–95, 2012

De Groot J, Tiberius R, Sinai J, et al: Psychiatric residency: an analysis of training activities with recommendations. Acad Psychiatry 24:139–146, 2000

Dobscha SK, Ganzini L: A program for teaching psychiatric residents to provide integrated psychiatric and primary medical care. Psychiatr Serv 52(12):1651–1653, 2001

Dobscha SK, Snyder KM, Corson K, et al: Psychiatry resident graduate comfort with general medical issues: impact of an integrated psychiatry-primary medical care training track. Acad Psychiatry 29(5):448–451, 2005

Druss BG, Zhao L, Von Esenwein S, et al: Understanding excess mortality in persons with mental illness: 17-year follow up of a nationally representative US survey. Med Care 49(6):599–604, 2011

Griffith JL, Gaby L: Brief psychotherapy at the bedside: countering demoralization from medical illness. Psychosomatics 46(2):109–116, 2005

Kates N: Sharing mental health care. Training psychiatry residents to work with primary care physicians. Psychosomatics 41(1):53–57, 2000

Katon WJ, Lin EH, Von Korff M, et al: Collaborative care for patients with depression and chronic illnesses. N Engl J Med 363(27):2611–2620, 2010

Kroenke K, Spitzer RL, Williams JB: The PHQ-9: validity of a brief depression severity measure. J Gen Intern Med 16(9):606–613, 2001

Mitchell P, Wynia M, Golden R, et al: Core Principles & Values of Effective Team-Based Health Care. Discussion Paper. Washington, DC, Institute of Medicine, 2012. Available at: https://www.nationalahec.org/pdfs/VSRT-Team-Based-Care-Principles-values.pdf. Accessed December 21, 2013.

Onate J, Hales R, McCarron R, et al: A novel approach to medicine training for psychiatry residents. Acad Psychiatry 32(6):518–520, 2008

Peek CJ, The National Integration Academy Council: Lexicon for Behavioral Health and Primary Care Integration: Concepts and Definitions Developed by Expert Consensus. Rockville, MD, Agency for Healthcare Research and Quality, 2013. Available at: http://integrationacademy.ahrq.gov/sites/default/files/Lexicon.pdf. Accessed December 21, 2013.

Raney L: The evolving role of psychiatry in the era of health care reform. Psychiatr Serv 64(11):1076–1078, 2013

Ranz JM, Weinberg M, Arbuckle MR, et al: A four factor model of systems-based practices in psychiatry. Acad Psychiatry 36(6):473–478, 2012

Rohrbaugh RM, Felker B, Kosten T: The VA psychiatry-primary care education initiative. Acad Psychiatry 33(1):31–36, 2009

Scharf DM, Eberhart NK, Schmidt N, et al: Integrating primary care into community behavioral health settings: programs and early implementation experiences. Psychiatr Serv 64(7):660–665, 2013

Shaw D, Blue A: Should psychiatry champion interprofessional education? Acad Psychiatry 36(3):163–166, 2012

Unützer J, Katon W, Callahan CM, et al: Collaborative-care management of late-life depression in the primary care setting. JAMA 288(22):2836–2845, 2002

Unützer J, Chan YF, Hafer E, et al: Quality improvement with pay-for-performance incentives in integrated behavioral health care. Am J Public Health 102(6):e41–e45, 2012

Varkey P, Reller MK, Resar RK: Basics of quality improvement in health care. Mayo Clin Proc 82(6):735–739, 2007

Wagner EH, Austin BT, Von Korff M: Organizing care for patients with chronic illness. Milbank Q 74(4):511–544, 1996

Wang PS, Lane M, Olfson M, et al: Twelve-month use of mental health services in the United States: results from the National Comorbidity Survey Replication. Arch Gen Psychiatry 62(6):629–640, 2005

Wright MT: Training psychiatrists in nonpsychiatric medicine: what do our patients and our profession need? Acad Psychiatry 33(3):181–186, 2009

Yudkowsky R, Schwartz A: Content, culture, and context: determinants of quality in psychiatry residency programs. Acad Med 75(10 suppl):S99–S101, 2000

Section II

Primary Care in Behavioral Health Settings

CHAPTER 7

The Case for Primary Care in Public Mental Health Settings

Martha C. Ward, M.D.

Benjamin G. Druss, M.D., M.P.H.

The reduced life expectancy of individuals with serious mental illness (SMI) has been noted since the 1800s (Dembling et al. 1999). Accidental causes were initially thought to explain the mortality gap, with experts focusing on suicide and other violent death as late as 1985 (Black et al. 1985). However, increasing evidence has emerged in the last two decades linking psychiatric and medical illness as the primary cause of excess mortality.

The interaction between medical and mental comorbidities is complex, and the mortality gap between those with SMI and the general population continues to widen. Meaningful changes in early mortality for patients with SMI will require programs that address a multitude of contributing factors, including maladaptive health behaviors, such as substance use and poor diet; adverse social determinants of health; symptoms of mental illness that interfere with medical treatment; metabolic effects of psychotropic medications; and poor quality of medical care.

Because persons with SMI are more likely to receive care through outpatient mental health centers than through primary care, these centers will be essential in addressing medical comorbidities (Alakeson and Frank 2010). Psychiatrists, with their combined medical and psychiatric training, are uniquely qualified to lead this effort.

SCOPE OF THE PROBLEM: MEDICAL MORBIDITY AND MORTALITY

Medical illness is highly prevalent in individuals with psychiatric disorders: more than 68% of adults with mental illness were found to have at least one medical disorder in the 2001–2003 National Comorbidity Survey Replication (Alegria et al. 2003). Rates of disease in those with SMI exceed those of the general population in every disease category (Parks et al. 2006). Specifically, patients with SMI display greater rates of obesity, diabetes, metabolic syndrome, chronic obstructive pulmonary disease (COPD), HIV, viral hepatitis, and tuberculosis than the general population. Cardiovascular disease (CVD) is also common, with prevalence increased twofold to threefold in patients with bipolar disorder and schizophrenia. CVD also occurs at a younger age in persons with SMI (De Hert et al. 2011).

When persons with SMI become medically ill, they experience higher standardized mortality rates (Table 7–1). Advances in treatment have greatly increased the life span of the general population, yet individuals with mental illness have lagged behind. This has resulted in a widening disparity, with premature death from natural causes contributing approximately 60% to early mortality in the population with SMI. The relative risk of all-cause premature mortality varies depending on the psychiatric diagnosis, ranging from 1.7 in major depressive disorder to 4.0 in some personality disorders (see Table 7–2). The magnitude of the mortality gap depends on the population studied. In a large, population-based sample (drawn from the National Health Interview Survey), those with any mental disorder died, on average, 8.2 years earlier than those without mental disorders (Druss et al. 2011). Patients with SMI treated in the public health sector are generally sicker and poorer and experience worse outcomes. A study in 2003 that gathered data from patients in the public mental health sector across 16 states found that people with SMI were dying, on average, 25 years earlier than the general population. Individual states showed even more dramatic results; data collected in Ohio from 1998 to 2002 demonstrated 32 years of potential life lost per patient (Parks et al. 2006).

MODIFIABLE RISK FACTORS

Natural causes are responsible for the majority of deaths in persons with SMI, and much of the excess mortality can be attributed to preventable risk. Modifiable risk factors that must be addressed in individuals with SMI include health behaviors, social determinants of health, medication effects, symptoms of mental illness, and quality of health care.

TABLE 7–1. Increase in standardized mortality rates for specific diseases in individuals with schizophrenia

Disease	Increase in mortality rate
Diabetes	2.7×
Cardiovascular disease	2.3×
Respiratory disease	3.2×
Infectious diseases	3.4×

Source. Adapted from Parks et al. 2006.

TABLE 7–2. Relative risk of premature all-cause mortality by diagnosis

Diagnosis	Relative risk
Major depressive disorder	1.7
Panic disorder	1.9
Alcohol use disorder	2.0
Schizophrenia	2.6
Bipolar disorder	2.6
Personality disorders	4.0

Source. Adapted from Eaton et al. 2008.

Health Behaviors

Adverse health behaviors have a huge impact on wellness. Four modifiable risk behaviors—tobacco use, substance use, poor diet, and lack of physical activity—are the cause of much of the morbidity and early mortality related to chronic diseases. Patients with SMI engage in these behaviors at higher rates than the general population, placing them at risk for chronic medical conditions and poorer outcomes (Druss and Walker 2011).

Tobacco Use

It has been estimated that between 31% and 44% of all cigarettes smoked in the United States are consumed by individuals with a diagnosable mental illness (Centers for Disease Control and Prevention 2013). This is partially due to the high rates of smoking in patients with psychiatric disorders; recent evidence shows that 44%–64% of individuals with SMI smoke, though prior data estimates indicated that the prevalence of tobacco use was as high as 88% in individuals with schizophrenia (Dickerson et al. 2013). Individuals with mental illness also smoke at an earlier age and are more likely to progress from casual use to dependence (Breslau et al. 2004). Additionally, intensity of smoking is greater in those with SMI. Approximately 50% of patients with schizophrenia are heavy smokers, consuming more than 25 cigarettes per day (Ziedonis et al. 2008). Smokers with schizophrenia take more puffs per cigarette when compared to control patients, which explains why they have higher levels of serum nicotine and cotinine (a metabolite of nicotine) than control patients who smoke the same number of cigarettes (Ziedonis et al. 2008).

Persons with SMI experience direct medical consequences from this extraordinarily high rate and intensity of tobacco use. Prevalence of COPD (chronic bronchitis and emphysema) is higher in individuals with mental illness, particularly schizophrenia. It is also suggested that those with mental illness have higher rates of respiratory cancers than the general population (Compton et al. 2006). Tobacco use is a well-known risk factor for CVD, and smoking contributes to the increased risk of CVD in patients with SMI. Overall, tobacco-related conditions account for approximately half of all deaths in persons with schizophrenia, bipolar disorder, or depression (Callaghan et al. 2014).

Indirect health consequences of smoking are also problematic. Tobacco taxation has resulted in a significant increase in the cost of cigarettes in recent years. In the general population, this has been an effective deterrent. However, studies show that persons with SMI report tobacco use as a "core need" above food (Forchuk et al. 2002). Thus, many individuals with SMI, particularly those living on a fixed income, continue to spend a substantial portion of their money on cigarettes. One study estimated that those with SMI who live in a high–tobacco tax state spend up to 27% of their monthly income on cigarettes (Steinberg et al. 2004). Because of this, these individuals have fewer funds available to support healthy behaviors, such as exercising or eating fresh produce. Patients may even forgo needed medications instead of abstaining from buying cigarettes.

Cigarette smoking also affects the metabolism of certain psychiatric medications by inducing the hepatic cytochrome P450 1A2 isoenzyme. This can result in lower serum concentration and decreased effectiveness at doses that may be therapeutic in nonsmoking patients. Medications commonly affected include many of the antipsychotics, such as fluphenazine, haloperidol, olanzapine, and clozapine (Desai et al. 2001).

The association between tobacco use and the population with SMI is complex and multifactorial. It has long been hypothesized that nicotine ameliorates both positive and negative symptoms of schizophrenia. Studies show that nicotine may enhance both sensory gating and visuospatial working memory (George et al. 2006). However, clinicians must take care not to attribute too much causation to the "self-medication" hypothesis, because it may lead to insufficient attention to other possible etiologies and limit efforts addressing cessation. Tobacco addiction, as well as comorbid substance use and withdrawal, must be considered when addressing continued use of cigarettes despite adverse effects. Many psychosocial factors play a role as well. Persons with SMI are often unemployed, resulting in increased idle time and less time in activities where smoking is unacceptable. Other factors include low income, low education level, and being unmarried. Many individuals with SMI also live in group homes, where smoking is the norm (Ziedonis et al. 2008).

Other Substance Use

Like tobacco smoking, the prevalence of problematic use of other substances in patients with SMI exceeds that of the general population. In some urban centers, drug and alcohol addiction occurs in as many as 50% of all persons with mental illness (Hunt et al. 2013). These elevated rates persist across multiple psychiatric diagnoses. Carney et al. (2006) found that compared to those without mental illness, people treated for schizophrenia are 12 times more likely to be treated for alcohol abuse and 35 times more likely to meet criteria for illegal drug dependence. They reported even higher rates of alcohol and drug use in patients with bipolar disorder; these individuals are 20 times more likely to have problematic alcohol use and 42 times more likely to be dependent on illegal substances (Carney and Jones 2006). This information is consistent with earlier data collected in the Epidemiologic Catchment Area study, which reported that 47% of those with schizophrenia and 56% of those with bipolar disorder will meet criteria for alcohol or drug abuse at some point in their lives (Regier et al. 1990). Patients with posttraumatic stress disorder (PTSD) also have high rates of a dual diagnosis (co-occurring mental illness and substance use). One review found that 21%–43% of civilians and up to 75% of veterans with PTSD had a substance use disorder (Jacobsen et al. 2001). Among depressed patients, roughly 20% of all individuals have a dual diagnosis; among patients with anxiety disorders, 15% have comorbid substance use (Grant et al. 2004).

Furthermore, polysubstance use is common in persons with mental illness. Lambert et al. (1997) reported that 55% of dual-diagnosis patients with schizophrenia self-reported use of multiple substances. The same study demonstrated a clinician-reported lifetime prevalence of polysubstance use in 72% of patients. In a group of individuals with a diagnosis of either schizophrenia or bipolar disorder, Verdoux et al. (1996) reported a 48% lifetime prevalence of abuse of or dependence on two or more substances.

Those with SMI experience many direct adverse physical effects from substance use. A study of nearly 12,000 Medicaid beneficiaries showed that patients with psychosis and a substance use disorder have the highest adjusted odds for being treated for five of eight medical disorders, including heart disease, asthma, gastrointestinal disorders, skin infections, and acute respiratory disorders (Table 7–3) (Dickey et al. 2002). Misuse of substances can lead to poor self-care and decreased adherence to medications, including those used to treat other medical problems. Intoxication can lead to risky behaviors, such as promiscuity, that place individuals at risk for sexually transmitted infections. It can also contribute to psychiatric destabilization, with more frequent hospitalizations and an increased risk of suicide and violent behavior (Buckley 2006).

TABLE 7–3. Odds ratios of eight medical disorders among Medicaid beneficiaries with and without a psychotic disorder and a substance use disorder

Disorder	Patients with a psychotic disorder		Patients with substance use disorder and no psychotic disorder
	With substance use disorder	Without substance use disorder	
Diabetes	1.60	2.62	1.40
Hypertension	1.43	2.11	1.19
Heart disease	4.24	3.19	2.92
Asthma	3.29	1.99	1.73
Gastrointestinal disorders	2.82	2.28	1.66
Skin infections	1.97	1.49	1.56
Malignant neoplasms	1.90	2.05	2.10
Acute respiratory disorders	2.04	1.40	1.41

Source. Adapted from Dickey et al. 2002.

Poor Diet

Unhealthy diet contributes heavily to medical comorbidity in persons with SMI. Multiple studies document the macronutrient content of community-dwelling individuals in this population. Brown et al. (1999) examined the diet of 102 patients with SMI in England and found that study subjects ate a diet higher in fat and lower in fiber than the general population. In Scotland, McCreadie (2003) found that persons with schizophrenia (particularly males) consumed fewer servings of fresh fruits and vegetables than the general population. Study subjects consumed a mean of 16 portions of fruits and vegetables per week; the recommended target in the Diet Action Plan for Scotland is 35 servings per week. Patients in this study also consumed less low-fat dairy and more breakfast cereal than the general population. These results are consistent with studies done in the United States. Strassnig et al. (2003) compared the diet of 146 individuals with psychotic disorders to nutritional data collected from the general population in the National Health and Nutrition Examination Survey. They found that study subjects consumed significantly more total calories, carbohydrates, and fat than the reference group.

Poor diet is a major risk factor for obesity and likely contributes to elevated rates in persons with SMI (Compton et al. 2006); those with SMI have an odds ratio of 1.5–2.0 of being obese when compared to those without a mental illness (American Diabetes Association et al. 2004; Weil et al. 2002). The metabolic risks of obesity are well known and include insulin resistance, diabetes, and hyperlipidemia. It is an independent risk factor for death from CVD (Pi-Sunyer 1993). Obesity is also associated with sleep apnea, gallbladder disease, osteoarthritis, and certain cancers (Muntaner et al. 2004; Pi-Sunyer 1993).

Socioeconomic disadvantage has long been noted in patients with SMI and may at least partly explain the elevated rates of poor diet in this population (Muntaner et al. 2004). Fats and sweets cost considerably less than fresh fruits and vegetables: the energy cost (U.S. dollars/1,000 kcal) of fresh produce is 10 times that of vegetable oils and sugars. Refined grains, added sugar, and added fat are also highly palatable and associated with overeating. In addition, access to fresh produce is limited in areas of socioeconomic deprivation. Research shows that lower-income neighborhoods have more fast-food restaurants and convenience stores and fewer full-service grocery stores (Drewnowski 2009).

However, low socioeconomic status (SES) does not fully explain the poor diet of patients with SMI: when McCreadie (2003) compared the diet of persons with SMI with individuals in the lowest social class in Scotland, those with SMI still met fewer of the recommended healthy diet measures. Clearly, there are other factors that contribute. More individuals with SMI are unemployed and smoke cigarettes, both risk factors for unhealthy food consumption. Additionally, symptoms of mental illness, such as apathy in schizophrenia, may lead patients to consume unhealthy convenience foods (McCreadie 2003). Finally, environmental factors may play a role. Many persons with SMI reside in group homes, which may not include healthy choices in their set meal plans (Chafetz et al. 2005).

Lack of Physical Activity

Individuals with SMI also engage in less physical activity than the general public. This sedentary lifestyle has been documented in numerous studies and across multiple psychiatric diagnoses. Elmslie et al. (2001) polled patients being treated for bipolar disorder in outpatient care and noted that they engaged in less exercise at low-, moderate-, and high-intensity levels than age- and gender-matched control patients. Brown et al. (1999) noted that individuals with schizophrenia in England spent less time exercising than members of the general population of a similar age. Daumit et al. (2005) looked at exercise levels in persons with both psychotic and affective disorders in an outpatient clinic in Baltimore, Maryland. They found a higher prevalence of inactivity and a lower prevalence of recommended activity levels in those with SMI compared with matched control patients from the National Health and Nutrition Examination Survey sample. Patients with SMI reported walking as the most common physical activity, with lower prevalence of other moderate- to high-intensity activities (such as jogging, biking, and playing competitive sports). Individuals with SMI also participated in fewer active leisure habits, such as gardening and dancing.

Sedentary lifestyle very likely contributes to the high rates of obesity in persons with SMI (Compton et al. 2006). Compared with those that are physically active, patients who are sedentary have an increased prevalence of a number of chronic diseases, including diabetes, hypertension, and CVD (Richardson et al. 2005). Lack of physical activity is an independent predictor of mortality in the general population and combined with poor diet is the second leading cause of death in the United States (Brown et al. 1999; Daumit et al. 2005). Conversely, regular moderate exercise has been shown to improve health by increasing high-density lipoprotein (HDL) and decreasing development of hypertension, type 2 diabetes, and CVD (Daumit et al. 2005). Health benefits associated with physical activity occur even in the absence of weight loss (Richardson et al. 2005).

Many factors contribute to sedentary lifestyles in individuals with SMI. First, education may play a role. The population with SMI has a lower education level than the general public (Kessler et al. 1995). Physical activity correlates with education level in both those with and without mental illness. Studies of the general population show that exercise counseling occurs more frequently in individuals with a higher education level, and this may mediate the correlation. In addition, lower SES is associated with decreased physical activity in the general population (Friscella et al. 2002). Because patients with SMI tend to have lower SES, they may not be able to afford exercise clothes or equipment. Even walking requires appropriate shoes and a safe physical environment, and these may not be available to the poorest individuals. Social factors may also play a role. Daumit et al. (2005) found a strong association between social isolation and inactivity in persons with SMI. Peer influence likely also contributes, and group homes may promote a sedentary lifestyle (Compton et al. 2006). In addition, many psychiatric medications (particularly the neuroleptics and mood stabilizers) cause significant sedation. Finally, symptoms of mental illness itself may contribute to sedentary lifestyle. These include the negative symptoms of schizophrenia, such as apathy and lack of motivation, which are challenging to treat and often remain prominent despite remission of positive symptoms.

High-Risk Sexual Activity

In addition to the above-described adverse health behaviors, high-risk sexual activity contributes significantly to medical morbidity in those with SMI. Though a lower percentage of patients with SMI engage in sex, those that are sexually active often display high-risk behavior. In a study by McKinnon et al. (1996) of 178 psychiatric patients, only 52% had been sexually active in the preceding 6 months. However, among this group, 58% had not used condoms, 48% had multiple sexual partners (more than one partner in the previous year), and 30% had traded sex for money or goods. Another study of patients with schizophrenia showed similar results: 44% of patients were sexually active, but among this group, 93% used condoms intermittently or not at all, 62% had multiple partners, and 50% traded sex. In addition, 12% of sexually active patients with schizophrenia had partners with risky sexual behaviors (a history of HIV, intravenous drug use, or blood transfusion) (Cournos et al. 1994). These statistics take on even greater significance when compared with those in the general population; a 1992 survey of over 10,000 heterosexual individuals showed that only 7% had multiple sexual partners and just 3.2% had risky sexual partners (partners with HIV, intravenous drug use, or a history of transfusion or who were nonmonogamous or had hemophilia) (Catania et al. 1992).

High-risk sexual practices contribute to the high rates of hepatitis C virus (HCV), hepatitis B virus (HBV), and HIV in persons with SMI. Prevalence of HBV and HCV in those with mental illness is 5 and 11 times, respectively, that of the general population (Rosenberg et al. 2001). Rates of HIV in patients with mental illness range from 3.1% to 22.9%, depending on study methodology (Cournos et al. 2005). Prevalence of coinfection with HIV and HCV is also significant (Cournos et al. 2005). Comorbidity of mental illness and HIV or HCV leads to a poorer overall prognosis, and mortality rates of individuals with schizophrenia and HIV are higher than those associated with either condition alone (Cournos et al. 2005).

Severity of psychiatric pathology may predict high-risk sexual behavior, with particular symptom clusters closely correlated to specific practices. Having multiple sexual partners was approximately 3 times more likely in patients with positive psychotic symptoms, perhaps reflecting beliefs that override rational use of information. Trading sex was 5 times more likely in patients with high scores on the Positive and Negative Syndrome Scale Excitement Component. This is not surprising given that this symptom cluster includes high impulsivity. Trading sex was also correlated with schizophrenia and was 3 times more likely to occur with this diagnosis than with other Axis I diagnoses. Positive symptoms were not related to trading sex. Thus, some other hallmark of schizophrenia must explain the association (McKinnon et al. 1996). Given the lower SES of persons with schizophrenia, economic incentive may play a large role. The high rate of substance use in those with SMI (see section "Other Substance Use") likely contributes to the increased prevalence of high-risk sexual behavior. In the general population, trading sex is associated with drug dependence. Additionally, patients with SMI have been shown to have inadequate or mistaken information about risks for HIV (Cournos et al. 2005). Finally, individuals with SMI are an extremely vulnerable population, and rates of violence against this group are extremely high. Studies show rates of self-reported sexual abuse of 34%–38% in hospitalized women with SMI (Goodman et al. 1997). Thus, sexual assault may partially explain the high rates of HIV and viral hepatitis in this population.

Social Determinants of Health

Social determinants of health are the economic and social conditions that influence health status in individuals and groups. Commonly accepted factors include the following: the social gradient, or the correlation of SES with poor health; psychological stress, including that experienced at work; early childhood development; social exclusion; unemployment; social support networks; availability of healthy food; addiction; and safe transportation (Wilkinson and Marmot 2003). As discussed in the sections "Other Substance Use" and "Poor Diet," both addiction and access to healthy food choices contribute to medical morbidity in persons with SMI. Many of the other social determinants of health also play a part.

Exposure to early trauma is a risk factor for both mental and medical problems. Studies indicate a graded response between the level of childhood abuse, household dysfunction, and poor health. Moreover, increasing numbers of adverse exposures during childhood lead to a greater risk of depression and suicidality (Druss and Walker 2011). In addition to early stress, lifelong stress can lead to both physical and psychological problems. Lack of money for basic needs, overwhelming caregiving responsibilities, and conflict in relationships are strong risk factors for depression (Druss and Walker 2011). Chronic anxiety and the perception of a lack of control over life choices are also closely linked to poor physical health. The correlation between psychological stress and CVD is particularly well documented (Wilkinson and Marmot 2003). A common mechanism likely underlies the close relationship between stress and mental and physical illness. Altered immune function and chronic inflammation have been increasingly shown to play a role in multiple medical and psychiatric conditions (Druss and Walker 2011). Stress can also result in persistently elevated sympathetic nervous system and hypothalamic-pituitary-adrenal activity. This may have negative metabolic and cardiovascular effects, such as increased rates of hypertension, weight gain, elevated glucose, heart disease, and stroke (Schulz et al. 2012).

Chronic stress is more common in those with lower SES, and those with SMI experience a disproportionate amount of poverty when compared to the general population. Studies consistently show a direct and graded relationship between poverty and poor health outcomes (Wilkinson and Marmot 2003). This is partially mediated by adverse health behaviors and the effects of stress on physiologic systems. In addition, physical environment and living conditions play a role. Individuals in low-income areas have greater exposure to pollutants and toxicants, including polycyclic aromatic hydrocarbons, allergens, mold, and lead. Many factors may mediate these exposures. Inadequate garbage removal, location near traffic or transportation centers, inadequate ventilation, and poor building maintenance may all occur in low-income areas (Rauh et al. 2008).

The social networks of persons with low SES may also contribute to elevated rates of mental and medical disease. Poor social networks are associated with higher levels of depressive symptoms, as well as poorer outcomes in bipolar disorder and schizophrenia (Druss and Walker 2011). Lower levels of social support are also linked to increased rates of CVD and a risk of adverse cardiac outcomes that is 1.5 to 2 times that of the general population (Druss and Walker 2011). Additionally, those without strong social networks are more susceptible to pregnancy complications and have higher levels of disability from chronic illnesses (Wilkinson and Marmot 2003). Positive social networks are hypothesized to mediate health by buffering the effects of stress (Druss and Walker 2011). Additionally, positive peer influence can improve health behaviors (Chinman et al. 2000).

Medication Effects

Side effects of medications prescribed for patients with SMI contribute significantly to the poor health seen in this population. Weight gain occurs with many psychotropic medications, particularly the atypical antipsychotics. Though clinical trials show an increased weight gain for patients on all antipsychotics when compared to placebo, there is clearly a hierarchy of weight gain potential. Clozapine has the greatest risk, followed in descending order of magnitude by olanzapine, quetiapine, risperidone, amisulpride, aripiprazole, and ziprasidone (Megna et al. 2011). These effects are clinically significant, with an average of 12 kg gained in 40%–90% of patients on olanzapine and up to 31.3 kg gained on clozapine (Nihalani et al. 2011). Recently approved atypical antipsychotics appear to have more moderate weight gain potential, with asenapine causing 0.9-kg weight gain in the first 3 weeks of treatment and iloperidone associated with 1.5–2.1 kg gained (Nihalani et al. 2011).

Medications used to treat affective disorders can also have an impact on body mass index. Mood stabilizers, particularly lithium and valproic acid, are associated with increased weight (Parks et al. 2006); 71% of patients taking valproic acid gain more than 4 kg; 20% of individuals taking lithium gain more than 6.3 kg (Nihalani et al. 2011). Antidepressants can also induce weight gain; 10%–20% of patients taking antidepressants experience treatment-emergent increases in weight, with an average of 1–3 kg gained. The tricyclic antidepressants are more likely to cause significant weight gain than the selective serotonin reuptake inhibitors (SSRIs), with an average of 3–4 kg gained on imipramine (a tricyclic antidepressant) (Nihalani et al. 2011). Mirtazapine is also consistently associated with more weight gain than the SSRIs (Nihalani et al. 2011).

Psychotropic medications often display complex pharmacodynamics, and weight gain is likely due to interactions with a number of neurotransmitters and neural circuits. Stimulation of serotonin$_{2C}$ receptors causes decreased food intake in mice, and those lacking these receptors become obese. Mirtazapine and many of the atypical antipsychotics (including olanzapine, quetiapine, and clozapine) are serotonin$_{2C}$ antagonists. Histamine may help to centrally regulate satiety, and psychotropics that block the H1 receptor are associated with greater weight gain. Additionally, anticholinergic properties of drugs may contribute to obesity, whether through sedation, direct appetite stimulation, or dry mouth leading to caloric fluid intake (Nihalani et al. 2011).

In addition to weight gain, atypical antipsychotics may cause other metabolic abnormalities. Both lipid and glucose abnormalities have been attributed to the effects of these medications. These metabolic abnormalities are mediated in part by weight gain, but they have also been found to occur independently of adiposity. Olanzapine and clozapine confer the greatest risk of dyslipidemia; quetiapine and risperidone confer intermediate risk. Atypical antipsychotics have the largest effect on triglycerides, but they also appear to raise low-density lipoprotein (LDL) and total cholesterol. Olanzapine and clozapine also are associated with the greatest risk of dysregulation of glucose homeostasis, including hyperglycemia and insulin resistance (Rummel-Kluge et al. 2010).

The major components of metabolic syndrome are increased central adiposity, elevated triglycerides, low HDL, hypertension, and impaired glucose tolerance. Metabolic syndrome is a major risk factor for both the development of diabetes and death from cardiac disease. The risk of developing metabolic syndrome is highest with use of clozapine, olanzapine, and chlorpromazine. One meta-analysis showed a prevalence of metabolic syndrome in approximately 50% of patients taking clozapine (De Hert et al. 2012).

The mechanism for metabolic abnormalities with atypical antipsychotic use is unclear. However, there does seem to be a dose-dependent relationship between metabolic abnormalities and atypical antipsychotics. Studies have shown correlations between the serum levels of olanzapine, possibly risperidone, and weight gain. Similar evidence has emerged concerning olanzapine and changes in serum lipid profiles (De Hert et al. 2012).

Psychiatric Symptoms

Psychiatric symptoms can contribute to the poor health of individuals with SMI. Disease recognition may be hindered by disorganized thinking, cognitive impairment, or poor insight. When patients recognize medical problems, amotivation or mistrust of providers may prevent them from seeking care. Symptoms may also make it difficult to navigate transportation and scheduling details that are necessary to access care. Once at the physician's office, disorganized speech or behavior may impede appropriate description of physical symptoms (Viron and Stern 2010). In addition, many chronic medical conditions require patients to maintain a self-care regimen. This may include taking medication regularly and engaging in lifestyle modification. Persons with depression often display low motivation and poor energy; those with schizophrenia frequently display prominent negative symptoms. Such symptoms likely interfere with treatment adherence. In fact, studies consistently show poor medication adherence in patients with depression or psychosis (Druss and Walker 2011).

Quality of Care

Though they carry a greater burden of physical illness than the general population, individuals with SMI receive lower quality of medical care. They receive fewer routine preventive services, including immunizations, cancer screening, and tobacco cessation counseling (Druss and Walker 2011). Many illnesses also go undiagnosed in persons with mental illness (McCabe and Leas 2008). Ultimately, this contributes to the extraordinarily high rates of nontreatment for chronic conditions. Data from the Clinical Antipsychotic Trials of Intervention and Effectiveness (CATIE) show that rates of nontreatment in patients with schizophrenia range from 30.2% for diabetes to 64.2% for hypertension to 88.0% for dyslipidemia (Nasrallah et al. 2006). Even when diseases are recognized, quality of care is inferior. In a study done at the Veterans Affairs (VA) Medical Center, diabetic patients with psychosis had lower odds of receiving diabetes standard-of-care monitoring (such as routine eye examination, as well as testing of hemoglobin A1c and lipids) (Parks et al. 2006). In addition, individuals with SMI and cardiac disease are less likely to receive angioplasty or coronary artery bypass grafts. After myocardial infarction, persons with SMI are less likely to receive drug therapies of proven benefit, such as beta-blockers, angiotensin converting enzyme inhibitors, and aspirin. This may help to explain why postmyocardial infarction Medicare patients with mental illness have higher mortality rates than the general population; after myocardial infarction, persons with schizophrenia are 34% more likely to die than those without mental illness (Newcomer and Hennekens 2007). Furthermore, during medical hospitalization, patients with schizophrenia are about twice as likely to experience iatrogenic complications, including postoperative infections and deep venous thrombosis (Parks et al. 2006).

The poor quality of care of individuals with SMI is partially explained by their decreased access to regular, continuous medical treatment. Persons with SMI underuse primary care services and overuse emergency and medical inpatient care (Mental Health America 2012). This is partially due to the structure of the current health care system in the United States, with treatment of mental disorders carved out from physical health plans. This fragmentation results in poor coordination of care between medical and mental health (Parks et al. 2006). In addition, finances contribute to this pattern of health care seeking. Those with SMI often lack adequate health care coverage; this has been cited as the most common barrier to receiving care (Druss and Rosenheck 1998). Patients with insurance still feel the financial burden of visiting a physician and are twice as likely to delay seeking treatment because of cost (Druss and Rosenheck 1998). Additionally, individuals who are insured may be unable to find a medical provider. Perhaps this is due to the high number of mentally ill patients in the public health system covered by Medicaid and the dearth of providers that accept Medicaid enrollees (Parks et al. 2006).

Health care structure and financial strain are not the only factors that hinder access to care for persons with SMI. Even in the VA system, where all veterans have coverage, individuals with schizophrenia underuse primary care services (Nasrallah et al. 2006). Symptoms of mental illness can lead to difficulty with keeping appointments and following recommended treatment plans (McCabe and Leas 2008). Psychosis and mania may also interfere with organized communication of medical problems with providers (McCabe and Leas 2008). In addition, patients with SMI may avoid medical care because of dissatisfaction with treatment. In one study, individuals with schizophrenia had an odds ratio of 1.37 of reporting dissatisfaction with the thoroughness of the provider and an odds ratio of 1.54 of reporting dissatisfaction with the provider's explanation of problems (Kilbourne et al. 2006). Many with SMI report that providers place too much emphasis on the symptoms of mental illness, such that medical concerns are not taken seriously (McCabe and Leas 2008). The legitimacy of these reports is confirmed by interviews with mental health care providers, who cite examples of general practitioners placing physical complaints secondary to psychiatric symptoms (McCabe and Leas 2008). Moreover, medical professionals report that they see mentally ill patients as disruptive and increasing the workload and decreasing the efficiency of the practice. Feelings of fear and frustration may lead physicians to withdraw from patients, impacting the quality of the service provided (McCabe and Leas 2008).

ROLE OF PSYCHIATRISTS IN ADDRESSING MEDICAL HEALTH

As discussed in the section "Modifiable Risk Factors," many interconnected factors contribute to the high rates of medical morbidity and mortality in individuals with mental illness. Changing the poor health of persons with SMI will require a creative and multidisciplinary approach. Psychiatrists are in a unique position to lead this effort, given that they are trained to treat both physical and psychological illness. Through collaboration with colleagues and further development of specific competencies, psychiatrists can effectively address each of the modifiable risk factors that lead to poor medical health in patients with SMI.

Adverse Health Behaviors

Substance Use

Because of the high prevalence of problematic substance use in individuals with SMI, it is likely that psychiatrists will treat a number of patients with dual diagnoses. Several organizations, including the VA, have stated that taking responsibility for substance use disorders is the standard of care for providers treating dual-diagnosis patients (Renner 2004). Fortunately, psychiatry has established more formal training in addiction than any other specialty. In addition to accrediting a 1-year psychiatry fellowship in addiction, the Accreditation Council for Graduate Medical Education requires general psychiatry residents to have a meaningful experience in addiction medicine. This includes a minimum of a 1-month curriculum that covers management of overdose, detoxification, maintenance pharmacotherapy, and behavioral interventions (Rasyidi et al. 2012). Many residency programs have expanded this requirement, with a focus on the longitudinal treatment of dual-diagnosis individuals in an outpatient setting (Renner 2004).

Because of this extensive training, psychiatrists, more than any other type of physician, should be familiar with both the pharmacologic and psychotherapeutic treatment of addiction. Several promising therapy modalities have been developed in recent years, including motivational interviewing, network therapy, and harm-reduction psychotherapy. Cognitive-behavioral therapy, with a focus on techniques such as relapse prevention, has also been proven efficacious (Renner 2004). Given the centrality of psychotherapy in the treatment of dual-diagnosis patients, collaboration with psychologists and other therapists may improve the effectiveness of psychiatrists in achieving positive outcomes.

Additionally, substance use disorders are associated with a number of serious medical consequences, including alcohol-induced liver, gastroenterological, and neurologic disease; stimulant- and alcohol-related CVD; and lung disease associated with marijuana and crack cocaine use (Rasyidi et al. 2012). Psychiatrists should, at a minimum, become familiar with these sequelae of addiction and learn to recognize signs and symptoms associated with addiction-related medical illness. Psychiatrists will likely need to work closely with primary care and subspecialty physicians to definitively treat these diseases.

Tobacco Use

Despite the relative expertise of psychiatrists in the treatment of addiction, tobacco cessation has largely been the work of primary care physicians. During clinic visits, patients with mental illness and tobacco dependence received smoking cessation counseling 38% of the time that they visited a primary care doctor but only 12% of the time that they visited a psychiatrist. Inpatient psychiatric facilities have shown even lower rates of treatment of nicotine dependence. In fact, an examination of multiple facilities revealed that less than 1% of all psychiatric inpatients were even assessed for smoking status (Ziedonis et al. 2008).

Given the high prevalence of smokers with SMI and the severe morbidity associated with tobacco use in this population, it is imperative that psychiatrists make every effort toward treatment. The National Institute of Mental Health cites many reasons why psychiatrists may be ideal providers of tobacco cessation treatment. First, patients already have a therapeutic alliance with their psychiatrists. Next, patients return regularly for mental health care even if not interested in quitting smoking, and quit attempts can be encouraged at each visit. Finally, smoking cessation counseling in mental health settings is relatively cost-efficient (Ziedonis et al. 2008). Additional reasons include the relative expertise that psychiatrists have in addiction and various modes of therapy, as well as their comfort with a combined psychotherapy/pharmacotherapy approach to illness.

However, psychiatrists must first adopt more proactive attitudes toward addressing tobacco use in this population. It is possible that the focus on nicotine as "self-medication" may have hindered recognition of patients' willingness and ability to quit. There is growing evidence that smokers with schizophrenia have high rates of readiness to quit. Additionally, quit rates for patients with schizophrenia are only slightly lower than those for the general population (El-Guebaly et al. 2002).

While outpatient settings have commonly been the venue for smoking cessation efforts, recent data suggest that inpatient units with forced abstinence may also provide an opportunity to assist patients with quitting. For example,

Prochaska et al. (2013) showed that engagement in smoking cessation treatment resulted in a rate of abstinence of 20.0% compared with 7.7% with usual care at 18 months after brief psychiatric hospitalization on a tobacco-free unit.

Both pharmacotherapy and psychotherapy have shown efficacy in smoking cessation for individuals with SMI (Compton et al. 2006). Chapter 10 ("Management of Leading Risk Factors for Cardiovascular Disease") addresses nicotine replacement therapy and other pharmacologic approaches to smoking cessation.

As with the treatment of other substance use disorders, psychiatrists may benefit from collaborative relationships. Psychologists and other therapists can be invaluable educators and consultants on psychotherapeutic modalities. Medical sequelae of tobacco use, such as COPD, are likely best addressed with the assistance of primary care providers. Promotion of environmental change, such as smoke-free clinics, will require psychiatrists to have good working relationships with facilities managers.

Diet and Exercise

Though somewhat controversial, increasing evidence is accumulating for food addiction (Fortuna 2012). Because of this, psychiatrists' relative expertise in addiction may give them particular skill in promoting a healthy diet. As with drug and tobacco dependence, assessing readiness to change and using motivational interviewing techniques may improve engagement. Specific behavioral techniques, particularly relapse prevention planning, may also improve adherence to dietary changes (Van Dorsten and Lindley 2011).

Outside the realm of addiction treatment, psychiatrists may employ many other evidence-based behavioral and cognitive exercises to help patients improve both exercise and diet. Self-monitoring of food intake and exercise is highly efficacious, and records can assist the psychiatrist in evaluation of current practices and areas that may need change. Other behavioral techniques include realistic goal setting, environmental changes, and stimulus control. Cognitive exercises, such as curbing unrealistic expectations and addressing negative thoughts, may also be helpful (Van Dorsten and Lindley 2011). Additional tips for diet and exercise counseling can be found in Chapter 10.

As with other therapeutic interventions, collaboration with psychologists and other therapists may improve efficiency and knowledge base for psychiatrists attempting to address diet and exercise. Dietitians can help motivated patients to make reasonable food choices. Certified peer specialists may also help model healthy diet and physical activity (Fricks et al. 2012).

High-Risk Sexual Behavior

As in the general population, those with SMI hold many false beliefs about the risks for HIV and other sexually transmitted diseases. Though not all data are consistent, several studies show a significant correlation between lack of information and high-risk behaviors (Cournos et al. 2005). Thus, education may be a good first step toward improving high-risk behaviors in patients with SMI. This may be done by psychiatrists in the course of a brief office visit when taking a sexual history. In addition, psychiatrists must be aware of the psychiatric symptoms that are associated with greater high-risk sexual activity. Studies show a link between high-risk sex and greater positive symptoms, more delusions, and higher scores on the "excited" symptom cluster of the Positive and Negative Syndrome Scale (Cournos et al. 1994; McKinnon et al. 1996). Not only should psychiatrists attempt to address these symptoms via pharmacotherapy, they may choose to specifically target this population for safe sex education and therapeutic interventions.

Though prevention is ideal, many individuals with SMI have already contracted sexually transmitted infections. Thus, psychiatrists should regularly test for HIV, HBV, and HCV in patients with high-risk histories. Routine use of a history-based risk classification system may improve consistency in this practice (Cournos et al. 2005). When HIV, HBV, and HCV are detected, psychiatrists should promptly refer patients for treatment, whether through primary care or directly to infectious disease and hepatology specialists. Coordination of care with these specialists is essential, given the clinical issues related to concomitant treatment of mental illness, HIV, and hepatitis. Antiretrovirals have been associated with the onset of psychotic and depressive symptoms in case reports, and interferon-alpha has been consistently linked with depression (Cournos et al. 2005). More frequent psychiatric evaluation may be necessary when using these medications. Additionally, there are many potential drug-drug interactions between psychiatric medications and antiretrovirals. Specifically, protease inhibitors interact with the hepatic cytochrome P450 system. The atypical antipsychotics and many antidepressants are metabolized through this system, leading to possible subtherapeutic or supratherapeutic dosing when combined with protease inhibitors (Cournos et al. 2005). Despite these potential complications, many patients with SMI have been safely and successfully treated for infectious hepatitis and HIV. Open communication with psychiatrists may allow medical specialists greater comfort with initiating these lifesaving medications in persons with SMI.

Social Determinants of Health

Psychiatrists may not realistically be able to change the adverse social determinants of health experienced by those with SMI. However, recognizing and addressing the effects of specific elements, including low SES and poor social networks, may make a great difference in the health of these individuals.

First, psychiatrists must use all resources available to decrease the impact of low SES on patient adherence to treatment. Physicians must be aware of the relative cost of medications, substituting low-cost or free medications whenever possible. Useful resources include the $4.00 formulary offered by many national chain stores, pharmaceutical patient assistance programs, and, in certain states, subsidized public health system pharmacies. Psychiatrists must also be aware of the costs of transportation and advocate for a central office location that is easy for patients to access. If feasible, psychiatrists may offer phone consultation or offer vouchers to offset the cost of transportation. On-site financial counseling or money management skills training, ideally provided by case managers, could also be helpful for patients with limited funds. Assistance in obtaining disability benefits and health insurance can also mitigate some of the financial problems.

Additionally, psychiatrists should seek to improve the social networks of patients with SMI. Psychiatrists should assess daily activities of patients and, when appropriate, make referrals to day programs. Involvement in peer-led organizations, such as support groups and clubhouses, should be strongly encouraged. Psychiatrists should also consider involving family members in treatment plans to improve support for the patients. In other underserved populations, including Latinos and African Americans, family involvement has been associated with improved treatment adherence and outcomes (Seo and Sa 2008).

Medication Side Effects

Psychiatrists must recognize and address the potential harm associated with psychotropic-medication prescribing. Monitoring for metabolic abnormalities is essential. However, even after the publication of screening guidelines for patients on atypical antipsychotics by the American Diabetes Association and the American Psychiatric Association, frequency of monitoring has changed very little. One study of over 23,000 patients taking atypical antipsychotics showed that testing for blood glucose and lipids at baseline, after publication of the screening guidelines, only increased from 17.3% to 21.8% and 8.4% to 10.5%, respectively. After 12 weeks of antipsychotic use, testing of blood glucose increased from 14.1% to 17.9% and from 6.8% to 9.0% for lipids (De Hert et al. 2012). Clearly, monitoring must be improved. Psychiatrists must establish and implement a standardized monitoring system, which can be based on the American Diabetes Association/American Psychiatric Association guidelines (Table 7–4). However, physicians must be aware that these guidelines describe a minimum of monitoring, and patients at higher risk should have more frequent testing. Patients with a personal and family history of type 2 diabetes, hypertension, CVDs, and smoking may require more frequent monitoring. Those with abnormalities on screening tests also merit closer follow-up. Finally, closer attention must be paid to individuals who are more susceptible to metabolic abnormalities with the use of antipsychotics, including those taking antipsychotic drugs for the first time, younger patients, and those with substantial weight gain.

TABLE 7–4.   Monitoring protocol for patients on second-generation antipsychotics

	Baseline	4 weeks	8 weeks	12 weeks	Quarterly	Annually
Personal/family history	X					X
Weight (BMI)	X	X	X	X	X	
Waist circumference	X					X
Blood pressure	X			X		X
Fasting blood glucose	X			X		X
Fasting lipid profile	X			X		X

Note.   BMI=body mass index.
Source.   Copyright 2004 American Diabetes Association. From *Diabetes Care*®, Vol. 27, 2004; 596–601. Modified with permission from The American Diabetes Association.

Furthermore, simply screening is not enough. Thoughtful prescribing must also be employed. Informed consent should include a discussion of metabolic risks of medications prior to initiation, and a plan to prevent weight gain should be included in the treatment. For certain antipsychotics (including clozapine and olanzapine), psychiatrists should aim to use the minimum effective dose and regularly attempt dose reduction when indicated. Polypharmacy should be avoided whenever possible; psychiatrists must be vigilant about examining medication lists at each visit to ensure that unnecessary medications are not inadvertently continued. If possible, medications with lower potential for metabolic disturbances should be used as initial treatment choices, particularly in patients with high-baseline cardiovascular risk. More than 75% of psychiatrists claimed in a nationwide survey that they would avoid prescribing a second-generation antipsychotic to lower the risk of metabolic disorders (Newcomer et al. 2004). However, these intentions weakly influence actual prescribing practices; data accumulated from VA providers show that antipsychotics with higher metabolic risk (including olanzapine, quetiapine, and risperidone) were prescribed to over 75% of patients with documented cardiometabolic disorders. Psychiatrists reported better efficacy, more or less sedating effects, and patient preference as the main reasons to continue to use these medications (Hermes et al. 2013).

When metabolic abnormalities arise, psychiatrists must advise patients to adopt lifestyle modifications. Multiple lifestyle interventions have been studied in persons with persistent mental illness. Though many studies show statistically significant results, the magnitude of effect does not equal that in the general population. Psychiatrists must address differences in the population with SMI to increase effectiveness of such interventions. As discussed in the section "Quality of Care," low SES and access to care must be taken into account. In addition, those with SMI often face cognitive impairment. Several studies of lifestyle interventions in patients with SMI have used techniques to combat such cognitive deficits. To improve initial comprehension, language was simplified and large font sizes were used in printed materials. To overcome low literacy rates, instructors read aloud and more visual materials were employed. Improved retention was targeted through the use of educational games, lesson repetition, frequent quizzes, and integration of mnemonic devices into modules. Providers called patients the night before classes, or gave participants calendars, to ensure that they remembered appointments (Cabassa et al. 2010). Psychiatrists may adopt some of these techniques to improve outcomes for individuals with SMI. However, physicians have had low efficacy when working in isolation to help patients with making lifestyle changes. This is due, at least in part, to time limitations in office visits. Formation of a multidisciplinary team, including nurses, dietitians, other therapists, and peers, may be invaluable in improving physician-led lifestyle modification programs (see further discussion of this in Chapter 8, "Providing Primary Care in Behavioral Health Settings," and Chapter 9, "Behavioral Health Homes").

When metabolic abnormalities persist despite lifestyle modifications, additional steps must be taken. First, psychiatrists may consider switching to a psychotropic agent with less risk. Many are hesitant to make medication changes in patients who are psychiatrically stable, and the risk of destabilization must be carefully weighed against the potential benefit to physical health. In patients who have gained more than 7% of pretreatment weight or have developed hyperglycemia, hyperlipidemia, or hypertension, physical benefits of switching drugs must be given strong consideration (De Hert et al. 2012).

If switching drugs is not possible, psychiatrists may want to consider adding medications that can counteract antipsychotics-induced metabolic abnormalities. Both metformin and topiramate have been shown to reduce weight gain associated with atypical antipsychotics (De Hert et al. 2012). Psychiatrists may also want to develop algorithms for the pharmacologic treatment of uncomplicated medical problems, such as hypertension and hyperlipidemia. If possible, psychiatrists may engage in consultative relationships with primary care physicians to assist with comanagement of metabolic abnormalities (discussed further in Chapter 10). When patients are more complex or consultation is unavailable, psychiatrists must not hesitate to make prompt referrals to family medicine, internal medicine, endocrinology, or cardiology to enable patients to receive appropriate care.

Access to Care

As discussed, individuals with SMI experience systemic barriers to care, including fragmentation of the medical system and low rates of insurance. In addition, those with SMI are disinclined to access primary care services even when they are readily available, as in the VA system. Mental health clinics are thus likely to be the principal connection that such patients have to the health care system. Because of this, psychiatrists may be the only physicians that persons with SMI encounter. Care for the physical health of these patients may, by default, fall into the hands of psychiatrists, and thus responsibility for the monitoring of all medical care is imperative to improving the health status of this patient population.

Psychiatrists may employ various models in order to meet the medical needs of individuals with SMI. Their level of involvement as providers of physical care can range from high to low. On one end of this continuum, physicians may provide truly integrated care by completing dual training in internal medicine or family medicine and psychiatry. However, this opportunity is currently limited to 39 available residency positions per year, spread across 19 programs. Yet even in general psychiatry training programs, there is a growing call to increase resident education in the treatment of common medical problems (Druss and Walker 2011). Psychiatrists may also gain more medical knowledge through elective rotations during residency, continuing medical education, or self-learning (see Chapter 10). However, many psychiatrists are not comfortable with taking on full responsibility for the physical health of their patients. In such cases, partnerships with primary care physicians may be preferable. In this model, services are colocated, with collaboration between internists and psychiatrists on a multidisciplinary team (discussed in Chapter 8). Patient-centered medical homes have been proven efficacious when organized in a primary care setting and are increasingly expanding to include behavioral health centers (Druss and Mauer 2010) (discussed in Chapter 9). For such projects to succeed, psychiatrists will have to increase their competency in consulting, managing, and working as part of a team. These skills are also essential in a facilitated-referral model, where mental health centers employ a case manager to improve linkage to selected primary care centers (Druss et al. 2010). This model depends upon the ability of psychiatrists to screen effectively for medical conditions and make appropriate referrals. Psychiatrists involved in these models must also use their liaison skills to educate internists and family practitioners about mental illness and thereby improve the relationship between individuals with SMI and primary care physicians.

CONCLUSION

Patients with SMI experience a heavy burden of medical morbidity and mortality. This is partially due to modifiable risk factors, including health behaviors such as smoking, problematic substance use, poor diet, low levels of physical activity, and high-risk sexual behavior. Social determinants of health also contribute to the poor physical health of those with SMI, with downward drift and low SES increasing stress and toxic exposures. Medication effects, as well as untreated psychiatric symptoms, also play a role. Despite the poor health of persons with SMI, quality of health care is also a problem.

Poor access partially explains the low quality of care that individuals with SMI receive. For many patients with SMI, psychiatrists are the only physicians that they will encounter. For this reason, psychiatrists must improve their ability to address the physical health of their patients. Fortunately, psychiatrists already have many of the skills needed to do this. In fact, their training in therapy and understanding of human behavior may make psychiatrists the best physicians to address modifiable risk factors. However, key competencies must be gained to optimize the ability of psychiatrists to provide quality medical care in the setting of behavioral health. First, more medical training is likely necessary. For those entering residency now, this could even include training in primary care. For those in current practice, optimum delivery of care will also depend on the use of evidence-based practices, such as multidisciplinary teams and patient registries. Developing leadership skills is essential to this endeavor, as is gaining an understanding of the health of populations and how to appropriately apply data. With appropriate training in these competencies and support from effective systems of care, psychiatrists can play an essential role in improving the life expectancy in their patient populations.

REFERENCES

Alakeson V, Frank RG: Health care reform and mental health care delivery (editorial). Psychiatr Serv 61(11):1063, 2010

Alegria MJ, Kessler RC, Takeuchi D: National Comorbidity Survey Replication (NCS-R), 2001–2003. Ann Arbor, MI, Inter-university Consortium for Political and Social Research, 2003

American Diabetes Association, American Psychiatric Association, American Association of Clinical Endocrinologists, et al: Consensus development conference on antipsychotic drugs and obesity and diabetes. Diabetes Care 27(2):596–601, 2004

Black DW, Warrack G, Winokur G: The Iowa record-linkage study, I: suicides and accidental deaths among psychiatric patients. Arch Gen Psychiatry 42(1):71–75, 1985

Breslau N, Novak SP, Kessler RC: Psychiatric disorders and stages of smoking. Biol Psychiatry 55(1):69–76, 2004

Brown S, Birtwistle J, Roe L, et al: The unhealthy lifestyle of people with schizophrenia. Psychol Med 29(3):697–701, 1999

Buckley PF: Prevalence and consequences of the dual diagnosis of substance abuse and severe mental illness. J Clin Psychiatry 67 (suppl 7):5–9, 2006

Cabassa LJ, Ezell JM, Lewis-Fernandez R: Lifestyle interventions for adults with serious mental illness: a systematic literature review. Psychiatr Serv 61(8):774–782, 2010

Callaghan RC, Veldhuizen S, Jeysingh T, et al: Patterns of tobacco-related mortality among individuals diagnosed with schizophrenia, bipolar disorder, or depression. J Psychiatr Res 48:102–110, 2014

Carney CP, Jones LE: Medical comorbidity in women and men with bipolar disorders: a population-based controlled study. Psychosom Med 68(5):684–691, 2006

Carney CP, Jones L, Woolson RF: Medical comorbidity in women and men with schizophrenia: a population-based controlled study. J Gen Intern Med 21(11):1133–1137, 2006

Catania JA, Coates TJ, Stall R, et al: Prevalence of AIDS-related risk factors and condom use in the United States. Science 258(5085):1101–1106, 1992

Centers for Disease Control and Prevention: Vital signs: current cigarette smoking among adults aged ≥18 years with mental illness—United States, 2009–2011. MMWR Morb Mortal Wkly Rep 62(5):81–87, 2013

Chafetz L, White MC, Collins-Bride G, et al: The poor general health of the severely mentally ill: impact of schizophrenic diagnosis. Community Ment Health J 41(2):169–184, 2005

Chinman MJ, Rosenheck R, Lam JA, et al: Comparing consumer and nonconsumer provided case management services for homeless persons with serious mental illness. J Nerv Ment Dis 188(7):446–453, 2000

Compton MT, Daumit GL, Druss BG: Cigarette smoking and overweight/obesity among individuals with serious mental illnesses: a preventive perspective. Harv Rev Psychiatry 14(4):212–222, 2006

Cournos F, Guido JR, Coomaraswamy S, et al: Sexual activity and risk of HIV infection among patients with schizophrenia. Am J Psychiatry 151(2):228–232, 1994

Cournos F, McKinnon K, Sullivan G: Schizophrenia and comorbid human immunodeficiency virus or hepatitis C virus. J Clin Psychiatry 66 (suppl 6):27–33, 2005

Daumit GL, Goldberg RW, Anthony C, et al: Physical activity patterns in adults with severe mental illness. J Nerv Ment Dis 193(10):641–646, 2005

De Hert M, Correll CU, Bobes J, et al: Physical illness in patients with severe mental disorders, I: prevalence, impact of medications and disparities in health care. World Psychiatry 10(1):52–77, 2011

De Hert M, Detraux J, van Winkel R, et al: Metabolic and cardiovascular adverse effects associated with antipsychotic drugs. Nat Rev Endocrinol 8(2):114–126, 2012

Dembling BP, Chen DT, Vachon L: Life expectancy and causes of death in a population treated for serious mental illness. Psychiatr Serv 50(8):1036–1042, 1999

Desai HD, Seabolt J, Jann MW: Smoking in patients receiving psychotropic medications: a pharmacokinetic perspective. CNS Drugs 15(6):469–494, 2001

Dickerson F, Stallings CR, Origoni AE, et al: Cigarette smoking among persons with schizophrenia or bipolar disorder in routine clinical settings, 1999–2011. Psychiatr Serv 64(1):44–50, 2013

Dickey B, Normand SL, Weiss RD, et al: Medical morbidity, mental illness, and substance use disorders. Psychiatr Serv 53(7):861–867, 2002

Drewnowski A: Obesity, diets, and social inequalities. Nutr Rev 67 (suppl 1):S36–S39, 2009

Druss BG, Mauer BJ: Health care reform and care at the behavioral health—primary care interface. Psychiatr Serv 61(11):1087–1092, 2010

Druss BG, Rosenheck RA: Mental disorders and access to medical care in the United States. Am J Psychiatry 155(12):1775–1777, 1998

Druss BG, Walker ER: The Synthesis Project: Mental Disorders and Medical Comorbidity. Research Synthesis Report No 21. Princeton, NJ, Robert Wood Johnson Foundation, 2011. Available at: http://www.mdhelpsd.org/downloads/medicalcomorbidity.pdf. Accessed May 10, 2013.

Druss BG, von Esenwein SA, Compton MT, et al: A randomized trial of medical care management for community mental health settings: the Primary Care Access, Referral, and Evaluation (PCARE) study. Am J Psychiatry 167(2):151–159, 2010

Druss BG, Zhao L, Von Esenwein S, et al: Understanding excess mortality in persons with mental illness: 17-year follow up of a nationally representative US survey. Med Care 49(6):599–604, 2011

Eaton WW, Martins SS, Nestadt G, et al: The burden of mental disorders. Epidemiol Rev 30:1–14, 2008

El-Guebaly N, Cathcart J, Currie S, et al: Smoking cessation approaches for persons with mental illness or addictive disorders. Psychiatr Serv 53(9):1166–1170, 2002

Elmslie JL, Mann JI, Silverstone JT, et al: Determinants of overweight and obesity in patients with bipolar disorder. J Clin Psychiatry 62(6):486–491, quiz 492–493, 2001

Forchuk C, Norman R, Malla A, et al: Schizophrenia and the motivation for smoking. Perspect Psychiatr Care 38(2):41–49, 2002

Fortuna JL: The obesity epidemic and food addiction: clinical similarities to drug dependence. J Psychoactive Drugs 44(1):56–63, 2012

Fricks L, Powell I, Swarbrick P: Whole Health Action Management Peer Support Training Participant Guide. Washington, DC, SAMHSA-HRSA Center for Integrated Health Solutions, 2012. Available at: http://www.integration.samhsa.gov/health-wellness/wham/WHAM_Participant_Guide.pdf. Accessed May 22, 2013.

Friscella K, Goodwin MA, Stange KCL: Does patient education level affect office visits to family physicians? J Natl Med Assoc 94(3):157–165, 2002

George TP, Termine A, Sacco KA, et al: A preliminary study of the effects of cigarette smoking on prepulse inhibition in schizophrenia: involvement of nicotinic receptor mechanisms. Schizophr Res 87(1–3):307–315, 2006

Goodman LA, Rosenberg SD, Mueser KT, et al: Physical and sexual assault history in women with serious mental illness: prevalence, correlates, treatment, and future research directions. Schizophr Bull 23(4):685–696, 1997

Grant BF, Stinson FS, Dawson DA, et al: Prevalence and co-occurrence of substance use disorders and independent mood and anxiety disorders: results from the National Epidemiologic Survey on Alcohol and Related Conditions. Arch Gen Psychiatry 61(8):807–816, 2004

Hermes ED, Sernyak MJ, Rosenheck RA: Prescription of second-generation antipsychotics: responding to treatment risk in real-world practice. Psychiatr Serv 64(3):238–244, 2013

Hunt GE, Siegfried N, Morley K, et al: Psychosocial interventions for people with both severe mental illness and substance misuse. Cochrane Database Syst Rev 2013, Issue 10. Art. No.: CD001088, DOI: 10.1002/14651858.CD001088.pub3.

Jacobsen LK, Southwick SM, Kosten TR: Substance use disorders in patients with posttraumatic stress disorder: a review of the literature. Am J Psychiatry 158(8):1184–1190, 2001

Kessler RC, Foster CL, Saunders WB, et al: Social consequences of psychiatric disorders, I: educational attainment. Am J Psychiatry 152(7):1026–1032, 1995

Kilbourne AM, McCarthy JF, Post EP, et al: Access to and satisfaction with care comparing patients with and without serious mental illness. Int J Psychiatry Med 36(4):383–399, 2006

Lambert M, Haasen C, Mass R, et al: Consumption patterns and motivation for use of addictive drugs in schizophrenic patients. Psychiatr Prax 24(4):185–189, 1997

McCabe MP, Leas L: A qualitative study of primary health care access, barriers and satisfaction among people with mental illness. Psychol Health Med 13(3):303–312, 2008

McCreadie RG: Diet, smoking and cardiovascular risk in people with schizophrenia: descriptive study. Br J Psychiatry 183:534–539, 2003

McKinnon K, Cournos F, Sugden R, et al: The relative contributions of psychiatric symptoms and AIDS knowledge to HIV risk behaviors among people with severe mental illness. J Clin Psychiatry 57(11):506–513, 1996

Megna JL, Schwartz TL, Siddiqui UA, et al: Obesity in adults with serious and persistent mental illness: a review of postulated mechanisms and current interventions. Ann Clin Psychiatry 23(2):131–140, 2011

Mental Health America: Position Statement 16: Health and Wellness for People With Serious Mental Illness. Alexandria, VA, Mental Health America, 2012. Available at: http://www.mentalhealthamerica.net/positions/wellness. Accessed March 20, 2013.

Muntaner C, Eaton WW, Miech R, et al: Socioeconomic position and major mental disorders. Epidemiol Rev 26:53–62, 2004

Nasrallah HA, Meyer JM, Goff DC, et al: Low rates of treatment for hypertension, dyslipidemia and diabetes in schizophrenia: data from the CATIE schizophrenia trial sample at baseline. Schizophr Res 86(1–3):15–22, 2006

Newcomer JW, Hennekens CH: Severe mental illness and risk of cardiovascular disease. JAMA 298(15):1794–1796, 2007

Newcomer JW, Nasrallah HA, Loebel AD: The Atypical Antipsychotic Therapy and Metabolic Issues National Survey: practice patterns and knowledge of psychiatrists. J Clin Psychopharmacol 24 (5 suppl 1):S1–S6, 2004

Nihalani N, Schwartz TL, Siddiqui UA, et al: Weight gain, obesity, and psychotropic prescribing. J Obes 2011:893629, 2011

Parks J, Singer P, Foti ME, et al: Morbidity and Mortality in People With Serious Mental Illness. Alexandria, VA, National Association of State Mental Health Program Directors Medical Directors Council, 2006

Pi-Sunyer FX: Medical hazards of obesity. Ann Intern Med 119(7 Pt 2):655–660, 1993

Prochaska JJ, Hall SE, Delucchi K, et al: Efficacy of initiating tobacco dependence treatment in inpatient psychiatry: a randomized controlled trial. Am J Public Health:e1–e9, 2013

Rasyidi E, Wilkins JN, Danovitch I: Training the next generation of providers in addiction medicine. Psychiatr Clin North Am 35(2):461–480, 2012

Rauh VA, Landrigan PJ, Claudio L: Housing and health: intersection of poverty and environmental exposures. Ann N Y Acad Sci 1136:276–288, 2008

Regier DA, Farmer ME, Rae DS, et al: Comorbidity of mental disorders with alcohol and other drug abuse. Results from the Epidemiologic Catchment Area (ECA) Study. JAMA 264(19):2511–2518, 1990

Renner JA: How to train residents to identify and treat dual diagnosis patients. Biol Psychiatry 56(10):810–816, 2004

Richardson CR, Faulkner G, McDevitt J, et al: Integrating physical activity into mental health services for persons with serious mental illness. Psychiatr Serv 56(3):324–331, 2005

Rosenberg SD, Goodman LA, Osher FC, et al: Prevalence of HIV, hepatitis B, and hepatitis C in people with severe mental illness. Am J Public Health 91(1):31–37, 2001

Rummel-Kluge C, Komossa K, Schwarz S, et al: Head-to-head comparisons of metabolic side effects of second generation antipsychotics in the treatment of schizophrenia: a systematic review and meta-analysis. Schizophr Res 123(2–3):225–233, 2010

Schulz AJ, Mentz G, Lachance L, et al: Associations between socioeconomic status and allostatic load: effects of neighborhood poverty and tests of mediating pathways. Am J Public Health 102(9):1706–1714, 2012

Seo DC, Sa J: A meta-analysis of psycho-behavioral obesity interventions among US multiethnic and minority adults. Prev Med 47(6):573–582, 2008

Steinberg HR, Hall S, Rustin T: Psychosocial therapies for tobacco dependence in mental health and other substance use populations. Psychiatr Ann 33:470–478, 2004

Strassnig M, Brar JS, Ganguli R: Nutritional assessment of patients with schizophrenia: a preliminary study. Schizophr Bull 29(2):393–397, 2003

Van Dorsten B, Lindley EM: Cognitive and behavioral approaches in the treatment of obesity. Med Clin North Am 95(5):971–988, 2011

Verdoux H, Mury M, Besancon G, et al: Comparative study of substance dependence comorbidity in bipolar, schizophrenic and schizoaffective disorders. Encephale 22(2):95–101, 1996

Viron MJ, Stern TA: The impact of serious mental illness on health and healthcare. Psychosomatics 51(6):458–465, 2010

Weil E, Wachterman M, McCarthy EP, et al: Obesity among adults with disabling conditions. JAMA 288(10):1265–1268, 2002

Wilkinson R, Marmot M: Social Determinants of Health: The Solid Facts. Geneva, Switzerland, World Health Organization, 2003

Ziedonis D, Hitsman B, Beckham JC, et al: Tobacco use and cessation in psychiatric disorders: National Institute of Mental Health report. Nicotine Tob Res 10(12):1691–1715, 2008

CHAPTER 8

Providing Primary Care in Behavioral Health Settings

John S. Kern, M.D.

The persuasive evidence for poor health outcomes for people with severe mental disorders is extensively summarized in Chapter 7 ("The Case for Primary Care in Public Mental Health Settings"). Because the integration of primary care within a behavioral health setting is of comparatively recent vintage, psychiatrists working on efforts to improve their patients' physical health will find that effective interventions are just now being devised. This chapter is intended to serve as a guide to these practices as they presently exist, focusing in particular on those that bring primary care services to adults with serious mental illness (SMI) in a mental health environment. While little definitive work has been completed so far, some effective forms of care and promising innovations have already been introduced for provision of primary care and supportive services to this population. It is hoped that this chapter will encourage and direct more effective psychiatric attention to patients' medical concerns.

STRUCTURE OF PROGRAMS

Programs intended to improve health outcomes in people with SMI generally include three major components: 1) primary care services made more easily available, often by bringing them to or near a behavioral health facility, 2) care management to assist patients in overcoming internal and external barriers to accessing needed primary care services, and 3) efforts to assist and encourage improvements in health behaviors. Programs vary in the means by which these components are provided and paid for and in the presence of additional supportive resources or sophisticated information management. Much of what follows will be a description of those additional components of care that may or may not merit duplication by those initiating new programs or updating those that have already begun.

Administrative Structures

A number of different on-the-ground funding arrangements have been made to support clinical models moving toward collaboration of primary care and behavioral health providers. Most existing programs have been initiated by community mental health organizations, which have reached out to existing or new primary care partners to create models of integrated care. A number of configurations exist, shaped by funding and administrative arrangements unique to each site. There are a number of variations, which may differ in degree of integration of clinical process or administrative structure.

Community Mental Health Centers and Federally Qualified Health Centers

The most common arrangement is a partnership between a community mental health center (CMHC) and a nearby federally qualified health center (FQHC). An FQHC may be invited to provide primary care services directly in a mental health center clinical site or through some facilitated arrangement in the FQHC site. The direct provision of service in the CMHC is viewed as preferable, given the difficulty for people with SMI in overcoming even apparently trivial barriers to accessing primary health services. This is usually funded by the FQHC applying for a "change of scope" to the Health Resources and Services Administration (HRSA), which permits primary care services to be billed at the favorable FQHC prospective payment system (PPS) rate. This funding advantage is enough to make such a program sustainable. In addition, it may be quite attractive to FQHC partners if there is access to a large Medicaid population, to which the prospective payment rate can be applied. These partnerships can be arranged to provide reciprocal services along the collaboration continuum, with the CMHC providing behavioral health services in the FQHC setting as described in Section I, "Behavioral Health in Primary Care Settings."

Federally Qualified Health Centers

An FQHC is a primary care clinic funded through the federal government as part of a program to improve health care access in medically underserved areas. HRSA is the federal agency responsible for oversight of this project. HRSA requires FQHCs to provide an array of services not often available in medically underserved areas, including obstetrics/gynecology, specialty pediatrics, urgent care, dental, and behavioral health services. In return for provision of these services, and for offering services on a sliding-fee scale, the FQHC is provided with an annual grant (called a Section 330 grant) and with authorization to bill all Medicaid (and Medicare starting in 2014) services at the advantageous PPS rate, which bases reimbursement on the actual cost of providing services.

Primary Care Services Without an FQHC Partnership

In some settings, the CMHC does not have access to a partner FQHC and may decide to engage primary care providers (PCPs) directly. This offers the advantage of convenient access for clients but is financially problematic, because the augmented FQHC billing rate is not available and expanding the primary care infrastructure can be a challenge for organizations that have no experience in this area. This also will require the CMHC to apply for separate billing designation as a medical (nonbehavioral health) provider. Arrangements in which a CMHC contracts with a non-FQHC primary care clinic or individual provider suffer from the same financial disadvantages. Without access to the PPS billing rate, a financial loss for the service is certain unless other funding sources are available.

CMHC With FQHC Status

A small number of CMHCs have taken steps to attain FQHC status, most notably the Cherokee Health System in Tennessee. This is a useful arrangement to facilitate integration of behavioral health and primary care and offers significant funding advantages, for example, to bill psychiatric services through the FQHC prospective payment rate system. Ongoing access to FQHC status may be uncertain after the initial funding of a large number of clinics shortly after passage of the Patient Protection and Affordable Care Act in 2010. A similar goal of an integrated care provision has been met by preexisting CMHCs and FQHCs that have merged. A number of CMHCs are pursuing status as FQHC "look-alike" clinics, which permit access to many advantages of an FQHC through a less competitive application process. The PPS rate is available in this process, but the federal 330 grants for uninsured and indigent patients are not. The Excellence in Mental Health Act of 2014 will allow CMHCs to become Certified Community Behavioral Health Clinics starting in 2017, and care coordination for physical illness is part of the certification process. The PPS rate will be available for eligible services in these new arrangements.

Global Payment Systems

The Oregon coordinated care organizations (CCOs) system is a global system of funding for physical, mental, and dental care for Medicaid beneficiaries (Oregon Health Authority, https://cco.health.oregon.gov). A CCO is responsible for coordinating all behavioral, physical, and dental care for Oregon Health Plan members through collaborative relationships. There is a global budget for all care rather than a set rate or a "capitated rate" for each different type of care. The CCO has more flexibility to manage dollars in a way that pays for improved health rather than having to rely on approved billed services. Performance measurements for CCOs provide incentives for better care, and CCOs are accountable for addressing avoidable population differences in health care outcomes.

Self-Contained Systems of Care

The Veterans Health Administration, the Department of Defense, and private insurers such as Kaiser Permanente are examples of self-contained systems of care in which primary and behavioral care are provided through one funding stream, most often utilizing the same medical record. This arrangement lends itself to integration, and the Veterans Health Administration, for example, has three integrated care models at work (A. Pomerantz, M.D., personal communication, May 18, 2013). This flexibility allows them to assign staff based on how they would like to configure their integrated care services. For example, they can use internal resources to assign care managers a caseload of patients, assign patients with SMI to one of their internal primary care teams, or locate primary care services within their behavioral health settings without having to look for external partners such as an FQHC.

Creative Amalgams

Some organizations leverage multiple funding streams to provide medical care, such as the case of the Washtenaw County Health Organization, a public nonprofit organization created by the University of Michigan and Washtenaw County. It is a community mental health service program under the state Mental Health Code, the designated substance abuse coordinating agency under the Public Health Code, and a Medicaid Prepaid Inpatient Health Plan for a four-county region (Koster and Reynolds 2006). This program allowed case management linkage from the mental health agencies to local PCP partners.

Clinical Structures

Clinical programs providing primary care services in the mental health setting vary in the scope and intensity of services provided. Some set the goal of providing focused primary care services, directed at important metabolic goals, and this has been the direction of many of the Primary and Behavioral Health Care Integration (PBHCI) grantees, discussed more in detail later in the "Existing Program Examples" section. Others have set up comprehensive primary care organizations.

Primary Care

Actual provision of primary care services is done in the usual way, by teams including primary care physicians, nurse-practitioners, nurses, medical assistants, and administrative staff. Often some improvisation is required given that space must often be found in the behavioral care organization's existing building. The complexity of the clinical problems presented by a population with SMI means longer clinical contacts are the rule, and it is expectable to see some loss of efficiency and productivity of the primary care staff as a result. When contracting with primary care organizations, this needs to be anticipated because experience has demonstrated it can lead to difficulty in the ongoing relationship due to loss of revenue that accompanies the lower productivity.

Frequently added in the behavioral health setting are staff devoted to supporting care provision, such as care managers, wellness coaches, and peer counselors. These providers are responsible for supporting and organizing structured care for patients with chronic (usually metabolic) illnesses such as diabetes and hypertension. The clinical outcomes of this process are typically tracked with the use of a registry, which is a data collection and management tool. The registry is also used to monitor for patients who do not persist with treatment, permitting active approaches to engage such patients, in an effort to improve outcomes in patients who would not have come to treatment on their own or at least not very consistently.

Health Behavior Change

Special attention is paid to health care behaviors and attempts to improve them, including support for healthy eating, exercise, smoking cessation, relaxation, and stress management. These activities have not ordinarily been offered in the conventional (primary care) setting, at least in part because they would not typically be funded. The literature on improving health care behaviors and outcomes in populations with SMI, summarized by Bartels and Desilets (2012), is sobering, given, for example, the difficulty in accomplishing significant weight loss even with highly structured programs. PBHCI organizations have tried multiple approaches with this issue. Some have tried partnering with local agencies, such as the YMCA or local fitness clubs with reduced fees for program clients. Several have implemented the InSHAPE program, devised by Monadnock Mental Health Center in New Hampshire. This is a structured fitness program including regular measurement, social support, and attention to nutritional variables, which has been shown to improve fitness in populations of individuals with SMI (Bartels et al. 2013; Van Citters et al. 2009).

Other approaches to health behavior change have been tried. A number of agencies have initiated ongoing training in motivational interviewing, a modality of interaction with patients that has been shown to be effective in assisting them to mobilize a wish to change and to act on that wish (Rollnick et al. 2008). Some centers have used concrete reinforcements, such as bus tokens, for participants in wellness programs. Finding culturally competent ways to engage patients can be a challenge: for example, Asian Counseling and Referral in Seattle, Washington, has transformed their model of mental health recovery to one of a "wellness service," which feels more comfortable culturally to their clientele. Every day they have "Asian Zumba," with movement to music from one of their clients' many home countries.

Coordination of Care

Coordination between primary care and behavioral health providers appears to be a crucial part of improving health outcomes. The completeness of coordination often depends on how integrated the services are between two organizations. Some examples of integration include the following:

- Creating teams that are completely integrated, providing both primary care and behavioral health services in the same team, using the same medical record
- Case coordination meetings, or "huddles," involving members of primary care and behavioral health teams who meet briefly to discuss patients that are being seen that day
- Shared access to electronic medical records (EMRs) or registries across agencies
- Coordination by virtue of case manager or care manager outreach to the other organization or outside medical providers

---

Example of Coordination of Care Using a Huddle

It took us a few false starts before we were able to make huddles part of the culture. In the end, what worked was a fairly typical plan-do-study-act cycle. We began with a medical assistant–physician pair who we identified as being particularly strong in terms of their relationship and in terms of their openness to change. We asked them to meet for 5–10 minutes prior to each clinic for 1 week and discuss whatever they thought would be helpful related to the patients to be seen during that day.

D.M., PBHCI grantee, Massachusetts

Team Members

A care manager, typically a nurse with a physical care background, usually oversees the provision of primary care services. On his or her own, or as leader of a team, he or she maintains a registry of physical health indicators (e.g., glucose, lipids, smoking status, blood pressure, and weight/body mass index) and communicates the need for treatment adjustments to the primary care team, as well as coordinating care across multiple medical providers. He or she provides clinical direction to bachelor's-level case managers and other nonlicensed staff as well as providing direct services to patients, such as physical assessment, teaching on health issues, and linkage with the primary care system.

Case managers, usually bachelor's-level clinicians already working to support the care of individuals with SMI in behavioral health settings, may be the most critical part of the team, where the "rubber really meets the road" in terms of assisting patients. Tasks include maintaining benefits and housing, keeping appointments, and interpreting "medicalese" in the context of medical appointments for patients who have difficulty doing so themselves. Other emerging trends include training case managers so they can educate patients on basic medical issues, helping to decode insurance problems, assisting in the development of improved health behaviors, and assuming an array of miscellaneous problem-solving tasks.

Peers are defined as persons living with mental illness. They have played a central role in the PBHCI team in keeping with the notion that patients should play an important role in their own recovery and in supporting the recovery of others. Peers can be involved in individual and group approaches to improving health behavior, such as smoking cessation, weight management, and physical exercise. They play a vital role in activating clients to self-manage their illnesses (Druss et al. 2010). In addition, groups supporting a holistic approach to overall wellness have been developed by the Center for Integrated Health Solutions (www.integration.samhsa.gov); Whole Health Action Management is a curriculum for a peer support group to encourage resiliency and wellness through relaxation, healthy habits, and development of self-management skills. Training of peers in this curriculum has been implemented in most of the PBHCI sites (www.integration.samhsa.gov/health-wellness/wham/wham-training).

PCPs may be physicians, nurse-practitioners, or physician assistants providing direct medical services. In addition to direct medical service, the PCP can provide oversight of the primary care support team, offering consultation and assisting them with obstacles their clientele may face when interacting with the medical system. The PCP may provide education to all staff in basic health literacy to help case managers, peers, and wellness specialists in motivating patients to self-manage their illnesses. In addition, the PCP can look at the health of the target population by examining aggregate data from the above-mentioned registry to establish priorities and target educational efforts. Another task is to interface with other treating medical providers in the community when care coordination issues arise, which allows the PCP to advocate for patients on behalf of the team. Finally, the PCP offers a crucial service by providing consultation to psychiatric providers on the chronic medical issues of their patients with SMI, including support of psychiatrists who may be providing their own direct care of common medical conditions.

Current roles for psychiatrists in the behavioral health setting should already include supporting and motivating attention to health issues, using safer psychotropic medications when possible, and making sure appropriate physical screening (weight, blood pressure, smoking status, lipid profiles, and blood glucose levels) regularly occurs and that abnormal findings are addressed. The creation of closer linkages with the primary care world creates exciting opportunities to expand the medical role of psychiatrists, for example, raising the profile of medical issues and making this part of the core mission of the behavioral health organization (see Chapter 9, "Behavioral Health Homes," for a listing of core duties of psychiatric providers). Psychiatrists can play important roles in training nonmedical staff about medical issues because of their training in the full scope of medicine. Some psychiatrists have started providing basic treatment of common metabolic conditions, such as hypertension, diabetes, or hyperlipidemia, with retraining and support with PCP consultation and/or written protocols (Raney 2013). This is parallel to successful collaborative programs mentioned in Section I of this book ("Behavioral Health in Primary Care Settings"), in which a PCP treats behavioral health disorders in the primary care setting with the assistance of a consultant psychiatrist.

EXISTING PROGRAM EXAMPLES

Primary and Behavioral Health Care Integration

The most extensive and systematic approach to developing effective care for physical health problems in people with SMI has been the PBHCI program mentioned in the section "Clinical Structures." This Substance Abuse and Mental Health Services Administration (SAMHSA) grant program was initiated in 2009. This grant was limited to CMHCs and some other community-based behavioral health agencies, and applicants were required to create a link with a primary care partner. The type of primary care partner was not specified, and some grantees elected to provide primary care themselves.

The purpose of this program is to improve the physical health status of people with SMI by supporting communities to coordinate and integrate primary care services into publicly funded community mental health and other community-based behavioral health settings. By building the necessary partnerships and infrastructure to support this goal, the expected outcome is for grantees to enter into partnerships to develop or expand their offering of primary health care services for people with SMI, resulting in improved health status. (Substance Abuse and Mental Health Services Administration 2009, p. 3)

Recommended components of PBHCI programs were influenced by the Chronic Care Model (Wagner et al. 1996), the Primary Care Access, Referral, and Evaluation (PCARE) study (Druss et al. 2010), the Improving Mood—Promoting Access to Collaborative Treatment (IMPACT) model of depression care (Unützer et al. 2002), and the concept of the patient-centered medical home (American Academy of Family Physicians et al. 2007). They include the following:

- Performing regular screening and registry tracking/outcome measurement at the time of psychiatric visits
- Placing PCPs, nurse-practitioners, or physician assistants in behavioral health facilities
- Using a primary care supervising physician within the full-scope health care home to provide consultation on complex health issues to the PBHCI team
- Using nurse care managers within the primary care team to increase consumer participation and follow up with all primary care screening, assessment, and treatment services
- Using evidence-based practices developed to improve health status in the general population and adapting these practices for use in the behavioral health system
- Providing prevention and wellness support services (including nutrition consultation, health education and literacy, peer specialists, self-help/management programs)

PBHCI grantees are in 43 states, and as of 2014, there were 106 grantees. With a few exceptions, the grantees are CMHCs who have reached out to local PCPs, usually a local FQHC, to provide direct primary care services. They have set up a system of support for access to medical care and improvement in wellness behavior, with variations dependent on local resources.

A high degree of variability in local conditions demands creativity in using the available resources to meet program goals. For example, there are communities in which no partner FQHC exists, and centers must create their own primary care services or establish partnerships with local agencies or local academic organizations. There are communities that require approaches to special cultural or access needs, such as offshore Alaskan islands or places like Seattle, Washington, with large multilingual immigrant populations. Some centers that serve large populations of homeless individuals have to devote more resources to patient engagement. For centers covering large rural areas, patients may have transportation difficulties and may not reach the center as frequently as would be optimal. Finding ways to succeed with special populations in changing wellness behavior requires some unique solutions, some of which do not succeed the first time around.

Examples of PBHCI grantee programs

The following are several examples of PCBHI grantee programs:

1. A mental health center with a long history of successful programming with peers used a population of peers as wellness coaches to form the majority of their program staff. One wellness coach is assigned to each behavioral health treatment team. All wellness coaches are pursuing formal personal training certification.
2. Another center also has made extensive use of peers and did extra work to make peer services billable under Medicaid. They have continued to pursue grant support to solidify peer-run programs, including a fitness center and a relaxation room, which focuses on mindfulness practices.
3. A merged mental health and primary care agency made attempts to treat patients with SMI in their primary care clinics and found that patients usually preferred to be seen in the home mental health clinics if this was possible. Other grantees have also found this to be the preferred location for primary health care.
4. A computer interface was devised to solve the problem of separate primary care and behavioral health EMRs so that information from both could be viewed simultaneously. This had to be abandoned later because of information technology performance issues and lack of user acceptance, although their primary care and behavioral health programs still have access to each other's data directly.
5. One mental health center serves a largely homeless population in an inner-city area. They became an FQHC themselves and were able to create both primary care and behavioral health record keeping in a single EMR, which is often very difficult. They also use a mobile van to provide primary care services to patients who might not be able to come in otherwise. They team up with two other organizations that also have mobile services to coordinate care on a given day of the week at a local soup kitchen.
6. There is no FQHC for many miles, so a clinic brought in a physician trained in bariatric medicine to provide focused services for the fre-

quently seen problems with obesity in this population. This provider has been able to offer state-of-the-art consultation for obesity in their clinic.

Outcomes of PBHCI Programs

The RAND Corporation, evaluator for the PBHCI grant, has published two evaluations of the grant program, including data on program characteristics and reported barriers to the establishment of programs, as well as outcome data on the success of the grant programs in improving health outcomes (Scharf et al. 2013a, 2013b). These evaluations accessed demographic and program data for 56 of the now 106 grantees, and study of the clinical outcomes for three early grantees was funded.

The RAND Corporation found that grantees were able to build integrated teams and to provide services to a diverse clientele with high rates of need, albeit at numbers less than projected. There was significant variation between grantees in the implementation of different aspects of integration. There were challenges implementing evidence-based wellness and behavior change programs, smoking cessation and monitored exercise programs such as InSHAPE, for example.

There were mixed results in terms of physical outcomes. After 1 year of the program, the three PBHCI grantees studied showed greater patient improvements in diastolic blood pressure, total cholesterol, and plasma glucose than patients in control organizations, but this was not true for systolic blood pressure, body mass index, and hemoglobin A1c%. There was no clear evidence of improvement in behavioral health outcomes from participation in the PBHCI program.

Interpretation of these equivocal results is important, given the need to continue to plan effective interventions to address the physical health of populations with SMI. Scharf et al. (2013a, 2013b) felt that the study had some methodological limitations, because it was designed initially to study a much smaller population, and they discuss the study's limited statistical power. It appeared that the control sites had more provision of primary care than expected. In particular, the process of meeting regularly with patients with SMI to discuss and measure health issues turned out to be a very powerful platform for initiating change.

The high degree of variation between sites in terms of which parts of the array of interventions were implemented and how persistently they were implemented makes assessing any new best practices difficult. Data do not exist with regard to which centers were rigorously applying evidence-based practices and whether their results were better. Scharf et al. (2013a, 2013b) recommended that more rigorous existing evidence-based practices for wellness and behavior change should be applied, that more thorough outcome measurement should be carried out, and that programs such as health homes and collaborative health programs such as TEAMcare (Katon et al. 2010) should be used as models for successful outcomes.

Despite the mixed results outlined here, it appears that there is the potential of meeting the program goal to "improve the physical health status of people with serious mental illnesses (SMI) by supporting communities to coordinate and integrate primary care services" (Substance Abuse and Mental Health Services Administration 2009, p. 3). There has been an explosion of interest in extending primary care services to psychiatric populations during the years of the grant, as exemplified by the high level of interest in attending integrated care sessions at psychiatric meetings and the growth of state and federal initiatives to address these populations. A number of grantees plan to publish their data independently in the near future. In addition, the Health Outcomes Management and Evaluation (HOME) study sponsored by the National Institutes of Mental Health is under way to look at patients with SMI with at least one chronic medical condition, utilizing an integrated community care intervention. The HOME study, which is being conducted by Ben Druss, M.D., who led the PCARE trial, is evaluating specific health and financial outcomes and may lead to a future direction for improving the health status of patients with SMI (http://clinicaltrials.gov/ct2/show/ NCT01228032).

Struggles of PBHCI Grantees

Registry Development

The initial PBHCI request for applications called for each participating center to engage in the development of a "registry/tracking system for all primary care needs of, and outcomes for, clients with serious mental illness" (Substance Abuse and Mental Health Services Administration 2009, p. 10). There was an expectation that a Web-based product would become widely available, but the organizations expected to market these Web-based registries did not deliver, and, with a few exceptions, less useful paper or Microsoft Excel versions have had to suffice. This useful tool for organizing care of a population with chronic illness has so far been underused in this program because of this barrier.

Weight Loss

As noted in the section "Clinical Structures," significant health behavior change in SMI populations is quite difficult. This is underlined in the publication of results from a program for weight loss specifically designed for a population with SMI (Daumit et al. 2013), in which the findings were again quite modest. Participants lost a mean of 3.2 kg (7.0 lbs) by the end of the 18-month study, which is comparable to that seen in lifestyle-intervention trials in the population without SMI.

This level of success, or lack thereof, can certainly be discouraging when psychiatrists are regularly faced with patients who can be 100 lbs overweight. Though there are not yet data to support this, it appears that there are some individuals who do have dramatic weight loss, following either medication changes or decisions to significantly alter exercise and eating habits.

However, Bartels and Desilets (2012) point out in their review that comparatively small changes in weight can be metabolically significant and can lead to significant improvements in health status. For example, a 5% or greater weight loss for overweight or obese individuals reduces risk factors for metabolic disorders and cardiovascular disease. They find that programs likely to succeed with this population are of longer duration (3 or more months), combine a manualized education and activity-based approach, and incorporate both nutrition and physical exercise.

Tobacco Cessation

Tobacco cessation is another critical issue for the health of people with SMI, given that 80% of individuals with schizophrenia smoke and given the health implications of smoking (De Leon and Diaz 2005). Focused consideration of this matter is another needed addition to the work of the psychiatrist. Removing obstacles to tobacco cessation treatment, including lack of attention from psychiatric providers, addressing knowledge deficits about treatment options in the community, and engaging care management staff to support abstinence attempts can double the low rate of successful quit attempts (Stead et al. 2012).

Workforce Issues

Recruiting and retaining PCP and case management staff for integrated programs has been a challenge, especially for rural centers. Some PCPs will not be a good fit for work in a behavioral health setting; they are uncomfortable with treating the patient with SMI, the complexity of problems, and/or the slow pace of the clinical work. Organizations are encouraged to seek out PCPs with some enthusiasm and compassion for this population.

In addition, training and engaging behavioral health case managers to expand their scope of work into the medical realm, touted as a potential asset that CMHCs can bring to this endeavor, has been difficult because they may not see medical issues as being central to their work. Attitude change in this regard depends upon strong administrative support for the integrated care mission.

The role of psychiatrists in PBHCI programs has been less inclusive than it could be, given the ability of psychiatrists to move somewhat more comfortably along the primary care–behavioral health spectrum. Approximately 10% of the PBHCI project directors are psychiatrists, and only a fraction of these have primary responsibility for management of the grant program, as opposed to a figurehead role. A small number have identified the opportunity to transform and strengthen their systems of care and have led innovation in such areas as developing and improving the EMR, improving collaboration with other medical agencies, and transforming assertive community treatment teams into "hot-spotting" units focusing on the intensive care of individuals with both mental illness and severe (and expensive) chronic physical illness. Many psychiatrists in PBHCI programs who do not serve as project directors are enthusiastic and supportive of the mission, but not all. Psychiatrists should be leading these new models of care, given their advantages in training and medical background and their enduring relationship with patients, though to date relatively few have embraced the opportunities available to do so (Kern 2013). See also Chapter 9 for a discussion of the roles for psychiatrists in the health home.

Engaging Primary Care Organizations

FQHCs and other PCPs rarely view the augmented medical care of people with SMI as part of their mission. Engaging them around the business and clinical case for this work can be a challenge, especially when it becomes clear that providing these services requires extra time and patience and may be less lucrative than usual care of an outpatient population. In situations where the primary care partner is an FQHC and has access to an advantageous Medicaid reimbursement rate, the high rate of Medicaid patients in the behavioral health patients' payer mix may be very attractive. It may be easier to engage organizations where there is global funding and where the population with SMI clearly makes up part of a medically and financially high-risk population that the organization has to manage well to succeed financially.

Ongoing Funding Issues

Grants, such as the PBHCI program, are not scalable to support a sustainable model of funding of integrated health services for SMI populations. One alternate funding source could be Section 2703 Medicaid State Plan Amendments for health homes, funded by the Patient Protection and Affordable Care Act. In a number of states, psychiatrists are involved in efforts to advocate for these amendments, which may include patients with at least one serious and persistent mental illness as an allowable population. Funding must be used to provide six additional care coordination services, not direct primary care services, under this option (see Chapter 9). A number of states have existing Medicaid waiver programs such as 1915i that cover case management and skill-building services. Many of these case management services have over the years been appropriately directed at support of medical services, and this continues to be a useful source of funding. In addition, the expertise in negotiating the entitlement and medical systems that behavioral health case managers have developed over the years is useful in supporting primary care provision. Some community behavioral health organizations have been looking into engaging with accountable care organizations, and other globally funded and bundled-funding organizations, to bring case management and collaborative care expertise with the expectation it will help contain costs and improve overall health outcomes and "bend the cost curve."

Non–Primary Behavioral Health Care Integration Programs

The introduction of physical health services into behavioral health settings has not been limited to participants in the PBHCI grantee program. A number of organizations have seen the need for these services and have set them up, often at a financial loss. Two program examples are the following:

- Pittsburgh Mercy Health System opened their own small family practice clinic with one physician and one physician assistant, to serve the population with SMI. They also make use of a care manager and some consulting psychiatrist time. So far they have seen 1,500 individuals, of the 17,000 seen by the mental health organization annually. This continues to be clinically very useful but not self-sustaining, because they do not have access to the augmented billing rates found in partnership with an FQHC.
- In Deschutes County, Oregon, a partnership has been created between Mosaic Medical and Deschutes County Behavioral Health. Local concern was driven by the large number of deaths of individuals with SMI in the community in the year prior to establishment of the partnership. In this setting, Mosaic Medical, which is an FQHC, sends a physician to a clinic located at Deschutes County Behavioral Health. This is a focused clinic, with the main FQHC clinic eight blocks away dealing with more complex problems. In fact, they started without an exam table at the mental health center site. The psychiatrist and the PCP have their offices next door to each other and are easily able to huddle on an informal basis as needed.

PROMISING PRACTICES FOR PRIMARY CARE IN BEHAVIORAL HEALTH SETTINGS

Linkages Between Electronic Medical Records

Finding ways to access information from multiple EMRs is becoming more common and is part of the meaningful use criteria for EMRs. However, in a number of states, access to health information exchanges has been problematic. An example of some of the problems faced is in Indiana, where the Indiana Health Information Exchange in its bylaws explicitly excludes behavioral health organizations. The original reason for this is the complexity of 42 C.F.R. (Code of Federal Regulations implementing federal drug and alcohol information confidentiality law) applying to confidentiality of substance abuse treatment records, and this has unfortunately hampered efforts of PBHCI grantees to engage in these health information sources.

Registry Development

Registry development was a requirement for all PBHCI grantees. It was anticipated that relatively convenient Web-based tools would be available to grantees, but unfortunately, this development has not occurred. It has yet to be seen what the additional benefit of a more sophisticated computerized registry will be for organizing chronic disease care in the behavioral health setting. Research completed on depression care using the IMPACT model has shown the effectiveness of this tool for the care of a population (Unützer et al. 2002).

Extending Care Management Competency to Behavioral Health Case Managers

The existing expertise of behavioral health case managers in assisting patients in improving their performance of activities of daily life and in interacting with bureaucracies of various kinds can be an invaluable asset in CMHC sites. The kind of community-based practical problem solving that is their stock-in-trade is exactly what is needed for people with SMI, who have to interact with a bewildering medical care system. There are some obstacles to the effective use of this modality. At the outset, behavioral health case managers often do not see their mission as including a high degree of attention to and responsibility for medical issues. They usually do not have the necessary medical knowledge required to be useful, for example, when interfacing between the patient, the medical office, and the PCP. This knowledge is crucial when supporting everyday functioning such as assisting the patient in a medication routine, keeping a blood sugar log, or attempting to improve the quality of the patient's diet. Training programs such as the case-to-care training offered by the SAMHSA-HRSA Center for Integrated Health Solutions are available to assist behavioral health case managers in learning some of these skills. This training is a start, but it has to be supported by the CMHC administration's ongoing embrace of primary care as a critical part of the CMHC mission. Whole Health Action Management (referred to in the "Team Members" section) is a related peer-supported health behavior change modality promulgated by SAMHSA.

Electronic Data Gathering

Electronic data gathering is a promising practice that provides a structured approach to managing population health in the behavioral health setting; it requires ongoing data collection and analysis to identify care gaps. There are some early attempts to streamline this, for example, by using handheld units or desktop computer kiosks to assist patients in self-entry of data such as depression rating scales.

Psychiatrists Providing Medical Care for Common Medical Conditions

Psychiatrists providing medical care for common medical conditions presents another innovative approach to improving the health status of the population with SMI. A collaborative approach between PCPs and psychiatric providers to address basic metabolic diseases is analogous to that of the IMPACT model for treatment of depression and is being explored. In this model, psychiatrists would follow and prescribe for such conditions as hypertension, diabetes, and dyslipidemias by protocol with the support of a consulting PCP (Raney 2013).

Consultant or Embedded Primary Care Provider

PCPs are an important addition to the behavioral health home in the Missouri and Ohio models at the time of the writing of this chapter. They oversee the primary health care of the identified population with SMI, supervise and educate the integrated team, and interface with the larger medical system in order to improve the quality of medical care provided to people with SMI. In addition, they provide a valuable partnership opportunity with psychiatric providers by joining forces to address the chronic health issues in this population. Chapter 9 describes the role of the consultant PCP in more detail in the example of the Missouri behavioral health home.

Typical Patient Care in a PBHCI Grant Site: Example

A patient presents to a scheduled psychiatrist appointment at the CMHC he has attended for years for the treatment of schizophrenia. He finds that now, before walking directly into the psychiatrist's office to see her, he is asked to see a medical assistant, who asks him who his PCP is and what his medications are and then proceeds to weigh him and take his blood pressure. He objects mildly—what does all this have to do with going to see his psychiatrist? The psychiatrist reviews the information; she notices his blood pressure is elevated at 160/90 and that unbeknownst to her, he has been taking atorvastatin and an unknown blood pressure medication prescribed by a local PCP. The medical assistant has checked to see whether routine monitoring of lipids and blood sugar has been done for this patient, who takes risperidone, and finds it has not been done for 22 months though it was ordered twice by the psychiatrist. After reviewing the patient's psychiatric situation, which appears to be stable, the psychiatrist walks the patient to the PBHCI nurse care manager and reviews the patient's medical situation with her, including that day's blood pressure measurement. The nurse care manager reviews the history of the patient's recent management of his blood pressure and talks to the patient and his case manager about communicating with his PCP about his blood pressure. The patient agrees that this is a good idea. The nurse care manager arranges an office visit with the PCP in the next few days and is able to clarify that the antihypertensive prescribed to the patient is lisinopril 10 mg daily. The nurse care manager enters this information into the SMI registry and sends a message to update the psychiatrist.

In the next couple of days, the nurse care manager visits the patient at home to check his blood pressure, finding that it is 175/96 at home. She notifies the PCP by phone, who increases the lisinopril to 20 mg daily, pending the patient being able to come in for an appointment. The case manager is able to arrange an appointment with the Medicaid office to have benefits reinstated. When the day of the PCP appointment arrives, the case manager phones the patient to remind him to get up in time for the appointment. He says that he doesn't really think he needs to go anymore, because he feels fairly OK and he doesn't notice any difference when he takes or doesn't take his lisinopril. She encourages him to come with her to the appointment anyway, and he agrees to do this, mostly because she asks him nicely. While they drive to the appointment, she educates him on his blood pressure, including the fact that it is usually asymptomatic, even though it is serious and needs treatment if it is regularly over the target of 140/90.

When they arrive at the PCP's office, the case manager asks the patient if he would like her to come in to the appointment with him. He agrees. When the PCP arrives, the patient cannot remember why the appointment was made. At the end of the appointment, after the PCP has decided to continue the new dose of lisinopril, the patient is given a written visit summary, including his diagnosis and treatment plan, medication information, lab studies needed, and information about nutrition and exercise. He and the case manager review this in the car on the way home.

A week later, the patient receives a phone call from his case manager, who calendared herself a reminder to prompt him about his follow-up appointment with the nurse care manager. When he arrives, he is weighed again and has his blood pressure checked, with a finding now of 136/84. The nurse care manager calls the PCP for a status report; they agree to continue monitoring him with the present treatment. As they talk, the nurse care manager realizes that in all the years the patient has been treated at the mental health center, no one appears ever to have asked him if he smokes, which he does, two packs a day.

The nurse care manager introduces the patient to a peer counselor trained in motivational interviewing, who invites the patient out for a walk (it's a beautiful day), and they start to talk about reasons why the patient might be interested in stopping smoking. "My blood pressure," the patient says. "That might be a good reason. And do you know how much these things cost?"

PRACTICAL TIPS IN PROGRAM DESIGN

The following practical tips are critical when designing a program:

1. *Be clear about the goals of the primary care clinic.* Depending on the size and complexity of a treatment system, the level and ambitiousness of integration goals may vary considerably. In some settings, a comprehensive primary care center will be part of the behavioral health facility. In others, the goal may be to do a focused approach to basic screening and care of basic metabolic issues, with more complex matters referred to a "home" primary care facility, hopefully one affiliated with the on-site primary care service.

2. *Think about devoting enough clinic space in the behavioral health setting.* Making the necessary room in the behavioral health organization costs money, and trying to run a program on a small scale can make it unsustainable for the primary care partner. For instance, 2.6 exam rooms per full-time PCP are considered an optimal amount of space in some primary care settings and having a one–exam room clinic in the CMHC would limit the PCP's ability to be more productive.

3. *Create an accessible and visible site.* Reports from PBHCI grantees suggest that proximity is critical in terms of the usefulness of the program and in terms of the likelihood that patients will make use of it. A number of grantees report that even going across the street to an FQHC partner is a significant obstacle to their patients.

Across the Street May Not Be Close Enough

We have been operating across the street from an FQHC for well over 20 years. We still needed the PBHCI program and imbedded primary care because a significant number of folks would never make the journey across the street. If they did, they often were not able to follow through with visits and recommendations, care was not coordinated or integrated, etc. It is so much more than the distance across the street. Integration is hard enough in our embedded programs—even side by side with behavioral health.

M.H., psychiatrist, PBHCI grantee site, Massachusetts

---

4. *Plan for unexpected financial issues.* Start-up costs may not have been considered in negotiations with a primary care partner. They may include making space and buying basic equipment and allowing time and money for expanding the program because of low utilization in the early days of operation. Considerable administrative work will be required to add authorization and infrastructure for medical billing. The number of behavioral health patients requiring physical health services may turn out to be less than the physical health provider expected, so it is wise to realistically forecast the number of clinic services required and plan for sustainability of what may be a small caseload, perhaps by making it possible for the primary care service to see a large number of their own patients from their home clinic at the CMHC site. From the point of view of a behavioral health organization's financial success, partnering with an FQHC to provide care directly at the behavioral health site is at present the ideal situation.

5. *Plan and nurture communication mechanisms.* Case conferences between staff to share information about patient care should take place on a regularly scheduled basis. These meetings might be viewed as expensive and time-consuming, especially for a large staff working on a rapid primary care timetable. They may focus on population care issues or high-need clients where strategizing is needed to optimize care. Less thorough but more focused is the huddle, which is usually thought of as a stand-up version of the case conference, hitting the highlights of which patients are expected today and what special interventions they may require. Even more spontaneous is the "curbside" consultation; these are unplanned, on-the-fly clinical discussions to share information or consult on cases. Less personal but just as important is communication between EMRs, often accomplished through a "tasking" function. Even if on-site, it is rare for partner behavioral health and primary care organizations to work from the same EMR. Some centers use software to pull information from both records to provide a working document with content from each. If the collaboration is off-site, it is important to identify staff responsible for and charged with facilitating communication, such as the nurse care manager.

6. *Use a registry to organize physical care of the psychiatric population.* EMR and registry functions supporting the chronic care model are what make population-based care possible. Some significant information services work may be needed to construct a registry in Microsoft Excel or Access or from within the EMR. Once created, there is a risk that the demands of everyday clinical work will derail attempts to manage a population, and the work required to maintain the registry will be viewed as of secondary importance. Referral tracking should be part of a registry function, but it requires significant care manager time. Without it, the actual percentage

of completed referrals to specialty care in populations with SMI appears to be extremely low. Linkage with case management outreach will also need to be an assigned task, as the funding and clinical supervision are likely to be separate. Demonstration of the positive outcomes that have followed from population management can help to motivate the extra work necessary to maintain these data collection instruments.

7. *Learn how to make health behavior change happen.* Really making a difference in health outcomes has to include patients changing their health behaviors. This has been a challenge in the PBHCI program, but it should be planned for in any kind of global care program. Training both primary and behavioral health staff in behavior change has to be planned, carried out, and supported. Educating on-site behavioral health staff about common medical conditions and training and supporting their use of motivational interviewing (Rollnick et al. 2008) will be an essential part of improving overall health care.

8. *Continuously reinforcing with the staff the need for integration is crucial.* Creating lasting attitude change in a behavioral health organization requires returning frequently to the subject of primary health care integration with staff to remind them that this is a permanent change in the mission of the organization. Looking for opportunities to demonstrate to behavioral health staff the positive impact that the program is having on patients can be a useful strategy, as is linking to wellness activities and initiatives that center staff may be engaging in.

9. *Make time for the psychiatric and primary care providers to collaborate on patient care.* Regular team meetings will foster mutual learning and trust and provide an opportunity for comanagement and shared medical oversight of this medically complex group of patients.

CONCLUSION

The best financial arrangement currently for providing primary care to the population with SMI is an FQHC-CMHC partnership. Locating primary care and behavioral services together is not enough. The use of care managers to coordinate care, using a registry to track data and treat to targets, and training behavioral health case managers to champion the cause of improving health are crucial to success. Sustaining programs requires keeping up enthusiasm over time for the mission, not getting discouraged by slow progress or the need to abandon projects that have not succeeded. It helps to show the larger mental health system that the interventions are working—with ongoing public relations and sharing data.

Psychiatrists bring unique expertise to both sides of the behavioral health/primary care boundary and unique credibility in terms of moving the mission of behavioral health facilities toward including physical care of chronic medical conditions. Psychiatrists can and should play an important role in improving the health of their patients with SMI, both by direct care and by leading the development of integrated systems of care. Psychiatrists need to seize opportunities to expand their roles from their current often limited position in the public sector. In addition to practicing psychopharmacology, they can move toward a central role directing the collaborative approach to medical and behavioral health problems, leading teams of caregivers caring for populations in a structured, data-driven process. This should enrich the psychiatrist's quality of work life while it provides an important key in improving access to and the quality of overall health care, both for the population with SMI and for patients overall.

Impact of Psychiatrist–Primary Care Provider Partnership

I was surprised at how working with a psychiatrist can help restore my idealism in primary care. After working with an SMI population for almost 20 years, I had slowly started to believe that I could no longer make a difference for the better in the lives of my patients. Working with a consulting psychiatrist helped me approach patient care in a more whole-person fashion and see beyond the numbers of blood work and blood pressure. It is restoring to work with someone that believes that the persons we serve can change for the better if we can come alongside them, listen, and help them to realize their goals. The psychiatrist is a tireless champion for those that society has rejected and forgotten.

T.W., PCP in CMHC setting, Pennsylvania

REFERENCES

American Academy of Family Physicians, American Academy of Pediatrics, American College of Physicians, et al: Joint Principles of the Patient-Centered Medical Home. Washington, DC, Patient-Centered Primary Care Collaborative, 2007

Bartels S, Desilets R: Health Promotion Programs for People With Serious Mental Illness (Prepared by the Dartmouth Health Promotion Research Team). Washington, DC, SAMHSA-HRSA Center for Integrated Health Solutions, 2012

Bartels SJ, Pratt SI, Aschbrenner KA, et al: Clinically significant improved fitness and weight loss among overweight persons with serious mental illness. Psychiatr Serv 64(8):729–736, 2013

Daumit G, Dickerson F, Wang N, et al: A behavioral weight-loss intervention in persons with serious mental illness. N Engl J Med 368:1594–1602, 2013

De Leon J, Diaz, FJ: A meta-analysis of worldwide studies demonstrates an association between schizophrenia and tobacco smoking behaviors. Schizophr Res 76(2–3):135–157, 2005

Druss BG, Zhao L, von Esenwein SA, et al: The Health and Recovery Peer (HARP) Program: a peer-led intervention to improve medical self-management for persons with serious mental illness. Schizophr Res 118(1–3):264–270, 2010

Katon WJ, Lin EH, Von Korff M, et al: Collaborative care for patients with depression and chronic illnesses. N Engl J Med 363:2611–2620, 2010

Kern J: Medical services, in Operationalizing Health Reform. Edited by Lloyd D, Lloyd S, Love R, et al. Washington, DC, National Council for Community Behavioral Healthcare, 2013, pp 53–78

Koster V, Reynolds K: Raising the Bar: Moving Toward the Integration of Health Care. Washington, DC, National Council for Community Behavioral Healthcare, 2006

Raney L: The role of psychiatry in the era of health care reform. Psychiatr Serv 64:1076–1078, 2013

Rollnick S, Miller W, Butler C: Motivational Interviewing in Health Care: Helping Patients Change Behavior. New York, Guilford, 2008

Scharf DM, Eberhart NK, Hackbarth NS, et al: Evaluation of the SAMHSA Primary and Behavioral Health Care Integration (PBHCI) Grant Program: Final Report. Rand Corporation, December 2013a. Available at http://aspe.hhs.gov/daltcp/reports/2013/PBHCIfr.shtml. Accessed May 20, 2014.

Scharf D, Eberhart N, Schmidt N, et al: Integrating primary care into community behavioral health settings. Psychiatr Serv 64:660–665, 2013b

Stead LF, Perera R, Bullen C, et al: Nicotine replacement therapy for smoking cessation. Cochrane Database of Systematic Reviews 2012, Issue 11. Art. No.: CD000146. DOI: 10.1002/14651858.CD000146.pub4.

Substance Abuse and Mental Health Services Administration: FY 2009 Grant Announcement: CMHS Grants for Primary and Behavioral Health Care Integration. Rockville, MD, Substance Abuse and Mental Health Services Administration, 2009

Unützer J, Katon W, Callahan CM, et al: Collaborative-care management of late-life depression in the primary care setting. JAMA 288(22):2836–2845, 2002

Van Citters A, Pratt S, Jue K, et al: A pilot evaluation of the In SHAPE individualized health promotion intervention for adults with mental illness. Community Ment Health J 46(6):1–13, 2009

Wagner EH, Austin BT, Von Korff M: Organizing care for patients with chronic illness. Milbank Q 74(4):511–544, 1996

CHAPTER 9

Behavioral Health Homes

Joseph Parks, M.D.

Many patients with serious mental illness (SMI) and substance use disorders are often seen more frequently by behavioral health specialty organizations such as a community mental health center (CMHC) than by other health care providers. As a group, these individuals have substantially higher rates of chronic medical conditions and premature mortality than the general population (Colton and Manderscheid 2006) and are less likely to receive adequate care for their medical conditions (Parks et al. 2006). Many of these individuals may be unable or unwilling to receive care in a primary care clinic, and even when they do, coordination between behavioral health and medical services may be poor (Druss and Walker 2011). For those individuals who have relationships with behavioral health organizations, care may be best delivered by bringing primary care, prevention, and wellness activities on-site into behavioral health settings (Parks et al. 2005).

The 2010 Patient Protection and Affordable Care Act (PPACA) established a "health home" (HH) option under Medicaid to serve enrollees with chronic conditions by building a person-centered system of care that achieves improved outcomes for beneficiaries and better services and value for state Medicaid programs (Mann 2012). The HH service delivery model is intended to provide a cost-effective, longitudinal "home" to facilitate access to an interdisciplinary array of medical care, behavioral health care, and community-based social services and supports for both children and adults with chronic conditions. HHs are designed to improve the health care delivery system for individuals with chronic conditions by employing a *whole-person* approach— caring not just for an individual's behavioral and physical condition but providing linkages to long-term community care services and supports, social services, and family services. The integration of primary care and behavioral health services is critical to the achievement of enhanced outcomes. The HH service delivery model is expected to result in lower rates of emergency room use, reduction in hospital admissions and readmissions, reduction in health care costs, less reliance on long-term-care facilities, and improved experience of care and quality-of-care outcomes for the individual. The guidance from the Centers for Medicare & Medicaid Services (CMS) regarding the Medicaid HH option indicates that HHs do not need to provide the full array of required services themselves, but they must ensure such services are available and coordinated (Mann 2010). This gives a behavioral health agency several options for how to structure the behavioral HH, depending on its resources (e.g., physical facilities, number of patients served, available workforce, financing options, community partners). This chapter will provide an overview of the HH model and a description of services and team members included in this approach to care and will examine the role of the psychiatrist.

A TALE OF TWO TITLES

The HH model described in this chapter was made possible by the PPACA (Public Law 111-148, as revised by Public Law 111-152), Section 2703, entitled "State Option to Provide Health Homes for Enrollees with Chronic Conditions." Section 2703 created a new section, 1945, within the preexisting Social Security Act (SSA; Section 1945). Because of this, it is referenced sometimes as Section 2703 and sometimes as Section 1945.

HISTORY

The medical/HH model was originally proposed by pediatricians and family medicine physician groups. In 1967, the American Academy of Pediatrics (Council on Pediatric Practice 1967, p. 77) proposed the medical home as "one central source of a child's pediatric records to resolve duplication and gaps in services that occur as a result of lack of communication and coordination." The American Academy of Family Physicians, American College of Physicians, American Academy of Physicians, and American Osteopathic Association wrote the "Joint Principles of the Patient-Centered Medical Home," stating that patient-centered medical homes should have seven characteristics: a personal physician; physician-directed medical practice; whole-person orientation; coordinated care; quality and safety; enhanced access; and adequate payment (American Academy of Family Physicians et al. 2007, p. 79). In 2008, the Department of Health and Human Services developed a conceptual model of the medical home, including service domains, training requirements, financing, policy, and research. It intended for the model to lower health care costs, increase quality, reduce health disparities, produce better outcomes, lower utilization rates, improve compliance with recommended care, and coordinate medical and social services required by the individual across the life span. The National Committee for Quality Assurance used this model to develop its medical home recognition program (Mann 2010).

State Medicaid programs have implemented delivery systems expanding on traditional primary care case management programs, many focusing on high-cost, high-user beneficiaries (not limited to specific diagnoses). While many of these models are physician-based, there is a growing movement toward interdisciplinary team-based approaches. Services such as care coordination and follow-up, linkages to social services, and medication compliance are reimbursed through a per-member per-month (PMPM) structure. Prior to the PPACA, states had already been using the authority in other sections of the SSA, such as Section 1932(a), and full-risk managed care plans and demonstrations approved under Section 1115 of the SSA to implement their medical homes. This new option offers the opportunity for behavioral health provider organizations to become HHs for the people they serve (Alakeson et al. 2010).

HEALTH HOME NAME NUANCES

Medical homes (also known as person-centered medical homes): This is a model for delivering primary care that includes the following: patient-centered care; comprehensive care, addressing physical and mental health needs, prevention, and wellness; coordinated care; accessible care; and a systems approach to quality and safety (Agency for Healthcare Research and Quality 2013). This model has evolved since 1967 and has had various funding mechanisms.

Health homes: Section 2703 of the PPACA allows states to amend their state plans (often referred to as State Plan Amendments or SPAs) to include integrated care models for individuals with chronic health conditions, including mental and substance use disorders. These HHs provide "person-centered, continuous, coordinated and comprehensive care." This model and its specific funding mechanism were created in 2010 by Section 2703 of the PPACA to expand the traditional medical home models to build linkages to other community and social supports and to enhance coordination of medical and behavioral health care in keeping with the needs of persons with multiple chronic illnesses. CMS expects HHs to build on the expertise and experience of medical home models, when appropriate, to deliver HH services.

SECTION 2703 REQUIREMENTS

The state option to provide HH services to Medicaid beneficiaries with chronic conditions became effective on January 1, 2011. Federal HH guidance lays out service requirements stemming from the PPACA and "well-established chronic care models" (American Academy of Family Physicians et al. 2007). The required services include the following:

- Each patient must have a comprehensive care plan.
- Services must be quality-driven, cost-effective, culturally appropriate, person- and family-centered, and evidence-based.
- Services must include prevention and health promotion, health care, and mental health and substance use and long-term-care services, as well as linkages to community supports and resources.
- Service delivery must involve continuing-care strategies, including care management, care coordination, and transitional care from the hospital to the community.
- HH providers do not need to provide all the required services themselves, but they must ensure the full array of services is available and coordinated.
- Providers must be able to use health information technology to facilitate the HH's work and establish quality improvement efforts to ensure that the work is effective at the individual and population level.

Selecting Patients: Eligibility and Enrollment

Individuals who are eligible for HH services must have at least one of the following:

- Two chronic conditions
- One chronic condition and the risk of having a second
- One serious and persistent mental health condition

"Chronic conditions" that a state HH model may select to focus on by statute include a mental health condition, a substance use disorder, asthma, diabetes, heart disease, and being overweight or obese as evidenced by a body mass index over 25. CMS can authorize (and has authorized) additional chronic conditions for incorporation into HH models. For example, Missouri HHs added developmental disabilities as a chronic condition to its HH state plan amendments. CMS also can authorize (and has authorized) state-proposed definitions of conditions and situations that constitute a "risk of having a second chronic condition." CMS also authorizes additional risks as proposed by states. Examples in Missouri include smoking and diabetes. Diabetes is classified as a chronic condition, and having diabetes includes the risk of a second condition, which means that like SMI, diabetes alone qualifies a person for a HH. The eligibility criteria are so potentially broad as to be able to cover almost all clients in a state's public mental health system.

Regardless of which conditions states select for focus, they must address mental health and substance use disorders and prevention and treatment services and consult with the Substance Abuse and Mental Health Services

Administration (SAMHSA) on how they propose to provide these services. States may apply to have their Medicaid state plan amended to include HHs, either in primary care, behavioral health specialty care, or both.

Health Home Service Definitions

Section 1945(h)(4) of the SSA lists six required HH services. CMS has not provided definitions of the six services but, instead, requires states to define each service, describe which team members are responsible for that service, and describe how health information technology will be used to deliver and support each service. States have broad flexibility to determine how to use health information technology in their HH models (www.medicaid.gov/ State-Resource-Center/Medicaid-State-Technical-Assistance/Health-Homes-Technical-Assistance/Approved-Health-Home-State-Plan-Amendments.html). An example of how Missouri defined these services is described in the section "Missouri Definition: Six Health Home–Required Services." These six services include the following:

1. Comprehensive care management
2. Care coordination
3. Health promotion
4. Comprehensive transitional care from inpatient to other settings, including follow-up
5. Individual and family support, which includes authorized representatives
6. Referral to community and social support services if relevant

Health Home Providers

The PPACA defines three distinct types of HH provider arrangements from which a beneficiary may receive HH services: designated providers, a team of health care professionals that links to a designated provider, or a health team. Examples of providers that may qualify as a "designated provider" include physicians, clinical practices or clinical group practices, rural health clinics, community health centers, CMHCs, home health agencies, and any other entity or provider (including pediatricians, gynecologists, and obstetricians) that is determined appropriate by the state and approved by CMS. Each designated provider must have systems in place to provide HH services and satisfy certain qualification standards.

Examples of the providers that compose a "team of health care professionals" are physicians and other professionals, which may include a nurse care coordinator, nutritionist, social worker, and behavioral health professional, and any professionals deemed appropriate by the state and approved by CMS. These teams of health care professionals may operate in a variety of ways, such as freestanding, virtual, or based at a hospital, community health center,

CMHC, rural clinic, clinical practice or clinical group practice, academic health center, or any entity deemed appropriate by the state and approved by CMS. The designated provider must have documentation evidencing that it has the systems and infrastructure in place to provide HH services and must meet qualification standards developed by the state and approved by CMS.

PAYMENT METHODOLOGIES

Section 1945(c)(1) of the SSA authorizes states to make payments for HH services, and the payment is for a team and not an individual provider. States have considerable flexibility in designing the payment methodology. States can structure a tiered-payment methodology that accounts for the severity of each individual's chronic conditions and the "capabilities" of the designated provider, the team of health care professionals operating with the designated provider, or the health team. They can also propose alternative models of payment that are not limited to PMPM payments for CMS approval. CMS requires a comprehensive description of the rate-setting policies in the Medicaid state plan and will judge the proposed method for consistency with the goals of efficiency, economy, and quality of care. While the PPACA specifically authorizes capitation payment for Section 2703 HHs, CMS has chosen to interpret its overall authority such that it will not allow true capitation payment (designated provider paid for every enrolled person each payment period) of a HH provider. CMS will only allow payment if the HH provider can document that the enrolled person actually received at least one of the six specific HH services during the payment period (commonly referred to as a case rate payment).

To provide an incentive for states to implement Section 2703, CMS includes a provision for an enhanced federal medical assistance percentage (FMAP) for HH services of 90% for the first eight fiscal quarters that an SPA is in effect. Thereafter, states can claim at the regular FMAP rate used for other Medicaid services during the calendar quarter. However, there is also a requirement that the eight quarters of 90% FMAP begin upon the effective date of the SPA. If there is a delay in implementation, this date could be different from the first day or first quarter when HH services claims are received. There is no time limit by which a state must submit its HH SPA to receive the eight quarters of 90% FMAP.

FEDERAL MEDICAL ASSISTANCE PERCENTAGE

Medicaid is a health insurance program jointly funded by the federal government and the states. The federal government's share of most Medicaid service costs is determined by the FMAP, which varies by state and is determined by a formula set in statute. The FMAP formula compares each state's per capita income relative to U.S. per capita income and provides higher reimbursement to states with lower incomes (with a statutory maximum of 83%) and lower reimbursement to states with higher incomes (with a statutory minimum of 50%). Certain Medicaid services receive a higher federal match.

DATA AND METRICS

HHs are required by CMS to track avoidable hospital readmissions, calculate cost savings that result from improved coordination of care and chronic disease management, and monitor the use of health information technology to improve service delivery and coordination across the care continuum. For the purposes of the overall evaluation, states are also expected to track emergency room visits and skilled nursing facility admissions. CMS requires states to calculate cost savings, preferably using a comparison group or, as an alternative, by constructing a precomparison/postcomparison of HH beneficiaries or an alternative comparison group of non-HH beneficiaries with similar chronic conditions and characteristics. Calculation of cost savings should include a tabulation of all Medicaid expenditures incurred for the HH group and the comparison group. CMS intends to at some time require a set of mandatory core measures. Until such time that CMS releases a core set of quality measures, states are expected to define the measures they plan to use to assess their HH model of service delivery. The measures are expected to capture information on clinical outcomes, experience of care outcomes, and quality of care outcomes specific to the provision of HH services.

EVALUATION OF HEALTH HOMES

The impact of the HH implementations will be examined in both an interim survey and an independent evaluation with reports to Congress. CMS requires states to collect and report information required for the overall evaluation of the HH model of service delivery. It is also a requirement that states collect individual-level data for the purposes of comparing the effect of this model across subgroups of Medicaid beneficiaries, including those that participate in the HH model of service delivery and those that do not. This evaluation, and the data gathered for it, will provide information that can help inform continued improvement of the HH models.

KEY PRINCIPLES OF THE EFFECTIVE HEALTH HOME

For HHs to work effectively, they must apply principles of quality care delivery (AIMS Center 2011).

Person-Centered Care

Person-centered care is the principle that all care should be based on the individual's preferences, needs, and values. In person-centered care, the patient is a collaborative participant in health care decisions and an active, informed participant in treatment. HHs provide an opportunity to transition from the traditional chronic model of illness to a recovery-based model in which health care providers help the people they serve have hope for the future (Substance Abuse and Mental Health Services Administration 2014).

Integrated Care

Individuals with mental health and substance use disorders, especially individuals with SMI, have significantly higher rates of comorbid conditions than the general population. When these chronic conditions go untreated, individuals often experience more serious physical illnesses that require increased medical treatment, such as costly hospitalizations (Parks et al. 2006). CMS requires that HHs have systems and processes to assure access to a wide range of physical health, mental health, and substance use prevention, treatment, and recovery services. The PPACA requires states to consult and coordinate with SAMHSA in addressing issues of prevention and treatment of mental illness and substance use disorders for individuals who are low-income and/or have one or more chronic illnesses; these individuals are at greater risk of developing mental health and substance use disorders. CMS and SAMHSA require states to coordinate with their state behavioral health authorities in designing their HH model and require that the behavioral health needs of individuals receiving services from a HH provider be addressed through a whole-person approach.

Evidence-Based Care

Evidence-based care is a core principle of integrating primary and behavioral health care and should guide care in behavioral HHs. It means using the best available evidence to guide treatment decisions and delivery of care. Care guidelines are the usual approach to condensing and summarizing all available research on a clinical problem. Embedding evidence-based guidelines in the routine provision of care through electronic medical records (EMRs), patient registries, and other computerized systems allows providers and consumers access to evidence needed for care decisions. Embedded decision flow charts for various conditions help users sort through the evidence-based treatment options and decide upon the best course of action. Finally, clinical decision support systems use data analytics to match a single evidence-based care recommendation out of a whole guideline to an individual's specific clinical situation. This prevents health care providers from having to memorize multistep guidelines or spend their limited time researching information on a specific condition.

Population-Based Care

One of the greatest flaws of current care delivery arrangements is that they typically depend on the patients alone to know when they need care and what care to ask for. One of the greatest changes that an agency must make to become a HH is transitioning from care that is driven by a series of individual patients' current chief complaints to care that is driven by analyzing the whole population served for care gaps and then using data analytics to select a group of patients with the most urgent care needs for the greatest opportunities for care improvement. Population-based care focuses on the health of an entire patient population by systematically assessing, tracking, and managing the group's health conditions and treatment response across the entire target group rather than just responding to the patients that actively seek care. Systems such as registries track the patient care data over time and can select for a particular condition, set of characteristics, practice/ provider group, or other parameter by actively and systematically assessing, tracking, and managing the group's health conditions and treatment responses (Halpern and Boulter 2000).

Data-Driven Care

Overall, HHs must change from the traditional way of thinking about the problems of the people they serve as a series of anecdote-driven activities to understanding the problems of the people they serve using explicit quantitative and qualitative analysis. It is a cultural change and work flow change not to be underestimated.

Data-driven care requires collecting, organizing, sharing, and applying objective, valid clinical data to guide treatment (Parks et al. 2008). The first step in HH development is to develop an inventory of potentially available data sets with individual demographic, health, and community status information and then develop a strategy for obtaining and integrating the available data sets into a relational database for program planning and individual care management (Druss and von Esenwein 2006). Because health care providers often do not have systems in place, or data available that allow them to determine utilization of services outside the agency, initial selection of persons to be enrolled in HHs is best done by the payer. There are two major sources of individual personal health information usually available for this initial analysis: payer patient claims information and EMR data extracts. There are advantages and shortcomings associated with both. Patient claims information has the advantage of providing a limited record of all care by all providers funded by that individual payer. Claims provide a record of all medications, emergency room visits, hospital admissions, outpatient visits, and specialty services, a record that includes the date of service, specific provider, diagnosis, specific identity code for each specific service, and type, dosage, prescriber, dispensing pharmacy, and days' supply of medications. They have the limitation of not providing important specific clinical values such as vital signs and laboratory results and do not include any health care situation that is not directly linked to a billable service (e.g., use of tobacco or whether a patient received a follow-up contact within 72 hours after admission). Claims also have the advantage of being in a standardized data format and aggregated database. EMR extracts have the advantage of containing much greater clinical detail, in particular vital signs and specific laboratory values. They have the disadvantage that each separate HH EMR has to be individually programmed to extract the data and then combine it into a single integrated database. EMR data extracts are also only available from practices willing to participate actively in care coordination. Most patients in HHs will be going to multiple providers, many of whom will not be providing EMR data. Therefore, EMR data provide much greater detail from a few providers but fail to provide any information from other providers.

HHs must develop the capacity to gather and aggregate data to use in three ways:

1. To develop a comprehensive picture of overall care received and current care gaps for each individual patient/client and all the patients served in the organization
2. To sort out which individual patient should receive immediate attention that day/week out of their total HH population
3. To track population-level improvement in both process and clinical outcome performance indicators both internally and in comparison with other health problems

The key data analytics tool is the patient registry, which is a database where key information about a target population is organized in one place. It supports the HH with information to increase the efficiency and effectiveness of care, maximize the outcomes for specific patient groups, and support the provision of population-based care. The HH clinical information system must be capable of organizing data on key subgroups of patients with particular conditions or characteristics, delivering reminders to providers, and providing feedback to clinicians. The data may include patient diagnoses, assessment or laboratory results, current and past treatment regimens, and appointments, which allows for the effective tracking of all the patients seen in the practice. Registry data must be sortable, allowing providers to select from a particular subgroup of patients or individual patients with specific treatment needs. Registries can identify subgroups of patients who are overdue for a follow-up appointment or necessary procedure. When set up in a format that allows multiple users to access it (e.g., a Web-based registry), a registry can facilitate communication and coordination of care across multiple health care providers and, when not all services are provided on-site, across organizations. The data can also be sorted by provider or by practice in larger systems, allowing organizations to evaluate performance and identify training needs. Some EMRs can be customized to provide a registry function or can be modified to allow for integration with an external registry.

CARE MANAGEMENT: PUTTING THE PRINCIPLES INTO ACTION

Care management combines the preceding principles in an integrated health care delivery work flow and entails following a defined population of patients to monitor their treatment response and adjust care as needed. Care management is a relatively resource-intensive strategy that is most effective when used with particularly complex patients with chronic conditions (Bodenheimer and Berry-Millet 2009). The care manager (CM) uses data to select patients with high utilization of avoidable services, such as emergency room visits and inpatient hospital admissions, and uses data to determine actionable care gaps to reduce this level of intervention in the future. The program enrollees are analyzed as a population to identify their common characteristics (e.g., particular diagnoses, comorbid mental health and substance use conditions, chronic pain, polypharmacy), which allows for identification of patient-specific actionable issues. Care management typically includes a health risk assessment, followed by educating patients about their conditions and how to manage them and recommended best treatments. The main work in care management consists of identifying care gaps and remediating them. Care gaps include not receiving a recommended preventive care screening, not monitoring laboratory results for the selected chronic conditions, not using best practice treatment for a chronic condition, nonadherence to medications, and lack of periodic follow-up with primary care or behavioral health care providers.

Within the HH team, the CM (often a nurse) utilizes the disease registry to monitor and identify gaps in care and then, working with the other HH team members, decides who will intervene regarding the identified problem. The CM or another delegated member of the HH team reaches out to the patient on a regular basis (often weekly at the start and then more infrequently as the patient begins to improve) to assess how he or she is doing, educate, and intervene as needed. The check-ins can be brief (usually 15 to 20 minutes) and can be conducted by phone or in person. Use of validated, standardized tools such as the Clinical Global Impression Scale or World Health Organization Disability Assessment Schedule 2.0 (World Health Organization 2012) to assess response to treatment is a best practice in care management. CMs use a registry as described earlier to keep track of their panel of patients and to make sure that they are followed up regularly.

The HH team, composed of the CMs, a primary care provider (PCP), and all the members of the traditional mental health treatment team, meets on a regular basis (usually weekly) and at the meeting reviews their panel of patients, prioritizes which ones present the greatest immediate need for care or opportunity for improvement, and plans for which members of the HH team will be responsible for specific interventions with those select patients. The selected HH team member conveys recommendations to the treating provider (could be a PCP or behavioral health provider), who then works with the patient to change the treatment plan and fix the identified care gap. This data-driven facilitated-referral approach has been proven effective in reducing Framingham risk scores and increasing utilization of preventive care (Druss et al. 2010a).

Care management functions can be done by different types of providers. The training and credentials of the CM will determine what functions he or she can appropriately and effectively manage, with more limited services being provided by those with less training. Historically, care management has mostly been provided by nurses and social workers (or equivalent master's-level professionals). Social workers are highly skilled at coordination activities, whereas nurses have more background in medical management and education.

Trained peers, community health workers, and health navigators (more often seen in the medical field) are increasingly being used to augment nurses and social workers in care management and for providing other wellness-related services. Community health workers have effectively provided screening, monitoring, patient education, and self-management support focused on chronic health conditions like diabetes and asthma (Goodwin and Tobler 2008). Peer support programs have excelled in patient engagement and empowerment (activation) (Druss et al. 2010b) because of the lived experience of individuals with mental health and substance use disorders when offering education and self-management support services (Salzer et al. 2010). Because these individuals have less training than nurses and social workers, the care management services they can provide will be more limited and must be overseen and their functions integrated with those of licensed CMs. However, they have the advantage of being lower cost than licensed CMs. Care management teams integrating both are likely to be more effective and have lower costs than either used alone. States implementing HHs will have to explain how HH care management is not the same as managed-care care management (see Table 9–1). CMS will not pay for the same thing twice.

TABLE 9–1. Apples and oranges: managed care and care management

Managed-care care management	Health home care management
Population: most are well most of the time	Population: all have multiple chronic conditions
Most have a few health care providers	Most have many health care providers
Primary focus: avoidable overutilization	Primary focus: inappropriate underutilization
Mostly communicates with providers	Mostly communicates with patients directly
Administrative relationship	Face-to-face personal relationship
Mostly e-mail, fax, or telephone communication	Mostly in-person communication
Intermittent contact by different care managers	Ongoing contact with stable team
Strangers working together	You know them and they know you
Provision of service not necessary to be paid	Provision of service necessary to receive payment

HEALTH HOME TEAM

The HH requires providers to work together as part of a multidisciplinary team that shares responsibility for addressing patients' comprehensive care needs. The team may be housed under one roof or function virtually, with members stationed in different settings. Regardless of location, it is essential that the members function as a single unit. Most behavioral health organizations implementing a HH care delivery model will already have multidisciplinary teams delivering behavioral health care. The HH team and behavioral health team should be the same team, not two separate teams, as the HH team is less likely to be effective when implemented as a separate service within the behavioral health organization. In most behavioral health organizations, this will mean adding at least a CM and other additional staff to the existing behavioral health treatment team. The membership of the team will depend on the individual's needs. For people with SMI receiving care in a behavioral HH, the team would consist, at a minimum, of their current psychiatric provider and behavioral health clinician (could be a therapist or case manager) and a PCP, who may be on- or off-site. It should also include the

CM, who tracks the individual's treatment response and coordinates care between team members, and may include a peer specialist, who provides wellness and recovery support, and/or a community health worker, who serves as a health navigator. Other providers such as a nutritionist, medical specialists (e.g., endocrinologist), a pharmacist, and other provider types may be involved based on the individual's needs. Regular team meetings and clear roles help the team establish which provider is responsible for what aspects of care and its coordination. In a behavioral health organization–based HH, the PCP, who may be a physician or a "mid-level provider" (e.g., a nurse-practitioner), plays a key role either as the provider of actual primary care services or in some models as a "consultant" within the HH team.

Different personnel could perform the team leader role, and they must be willing to take responsibility for assuring that the six core HH services are being delivered. The physician (or physician's delegate, such as an advanced-practice nurse or physician assistant) who has the most frequent contact with the patient would be an excellent choice for the team leader if adequate time and funding are provided to allow him or her to fulfill this role (lost productivity in the direct provision of behavioral health in exchange for a key role in improving the health status of the population with SMI). In many behavioral health organizations, this will be the treating psychiatric provider. It is essential that the team leader physician regularly attend the treatment team meetings and be available to the CMs. This requires that the psychiatrist now become involved with, and responsible for, the patient's general medical care to the same extent that he or she is involved with and responsible for his or her patients getting behavioral health community support services such as assistance with housing and employment. The team leader psychiatrist is not responsible for the actual provision and quality of primary and general medical care in a HH, but he or she is responsible for identifying that there are unmet needs (in this case general medical care) and ensuring that someone on the team is working to get those needs met. Ideally, a PCP works with the HH team to oversee the treatment of general medical conditions and review the registry data. The PCP-psychiatrist partnership creates an ideal platform for ensuring that the health care of patients with SMI receives high-level attention and intervention.

Case Example: Integration in the CMHC Health Home

Treating patients as a HH team benefits patients, psychiatrists, and PCPs. Dr. Day is both a PCP at an FQHC and a PCP consultant at a CMHC. Because Dr. Asher is a psychiatrist at the same federally qualified health center (FQHC) and CMHC, the two physicians collaborate on the care of many patients. One patient of the FQHC, L.R., was diagnosed with major depression. His somatic preoccupation and depression were so disabling that L.R. lost his job. Because of the loss of income, his housing was threatened. The PCP referred to Dr. Asher, who adjusted L.R.'s psychotropic medications and referred L.R. to the CMHC for case management. Dr. Day took over L.R.'s primary care and followed Dr. Asher's recommendation to see L.R. more often because of his disabling somatization. Because of depression treatment by Dr. Asher with simultaneous fibromyalgia treatment by Dr. Day, his Patient Health Questionnaire depression rating scale (PHQ-9) score decreased to below 10, he is more stable and independent, and he needs to be seen only infrequently now by his two physicians. When problems do reemerge, Drs. Day and Asher consult with each other because they recognize that the treatment of the whole patient requires a HH team.

The functions of the PCP in the Missouri HH are listed in Table 9–2 and can serve as a guide for other states wishing to include this important feature in the makeup of their team. The PCPs in the Missouri HH model are called "consultants," and in the Ohio model they are called "embedded" PCPs. Their functions are somewhat different. In Missouri, they guide the HH team but do not provide direct primary care service, whereas in Ohio they could do both (but SPA funding cannot be used for this direct provision of primary care services). The HH psychiatrist is in a position analogous to PCPs who, while not responsible for the direct provision of specialty medical care, are responsible for identifying when there is a need for specialty care and doing their best to see that that need is addressed. The roles of the HH psychiatrists are listed in Table 9–3, and they provide a nice example of how the psychiatric and primary care staff can have a synergistic relationship in their approach to taking care of patients. It is necessary for HH psychiatrists and CMs, who may be psychiatric nurses, to have access to PCPs and nurse CMs as members of the HH team in order to adequately provide the link to knowledge about general medical conditions in order to fulfill the responsibility of care delivery in the HH model. Models that rely solely on the medical knowledge of their existing psychiatric providers and psychiatrically trained nurses will lose this essential benefit.

The team works from a single care plan designed to address all physical health, behavioral health, and wellness needs. There should not be separate care plans for the HH and traditional behavioral health services, and the care plan is developed collaboratively with the patient. The plan should contain and integrate behavioral health goals, medical care goals, functional/rehabilitation goals, and wellness lifestyle goals to effectively facilitate recovery and wellness using a whole-person approach.

Teams usually meet weekly to review and discuss patients, typically focusing on those in treatment who are not responding well to the current care plan. Some teams start off each day with a team "huddle," in which the group reviews the patients to be seen that day. Communications can occur effectively and efficiently via an EMR or a registry. For teams working in an

TABLE 9–2.   Primary care provider consultant role in the Missouri health home

Establish priorities for disease management based on reviewing data. Identify patients who require immediate attention and select chronic diseases for intervention and initiatives that will have the greatest impact on the care of the population.

Provide education to both medical and nonmedical staff, the community, and patients.

Provide case consultation through regular team meetings with case managers, psychiatric providers, and other members of the health home team.

Develop collaborative relationships with psychiatric medical teams, external primary care providers, hospitals, and other community linkages to improve care.

Source.   From Parks et al. 2012.

TABLE 9–3.   Psychiatric provider role in the Missouri health home

Medical leadership and shared medical oversight:
  Psychiatric prescribers should provide leadership in the medical treatment of psychiatric disorders and share medical oversight with their primary care colleagues in the management of comorbid medical conditions. This includes medical treatment of psychiatric disorders, minimizing iatrogenic complications due to psychotropic medications, treating medical conditions by referral to PCPs or some limited algorithm-guided treatment in collaboration with the individual's PCP, and collaborating with the PCP by sharing laboratory results and treatment regimens to manage the overall health of each individual.

Collaboration with other team members in the comprehensive care management of health care home enrollees:
  Psychiatrists and psychiatric prescribers should collaborate with the other health care home team members in promoting recovery from serious mental illness, the self-management of other chronic medical conditions, and the adoption of healthy lifestyles. This includes participation in team meetings to plan the overall treatment, counseling individuals regarding lifestyle modifications, developing comprehensive care management strategies for individuals with complex medical/behavioral needs, engaging with the PCPs to improve each other's ability to "see the whole person" by exchange of information, and championing behavioral health expertise in support of behavior change.

Note.   PCP=primary care provider.
Source.   From Parks et al. 2013.

agency without an EMR or registry, faxes, encrypted e-mails, and secure online shared documents can facilitate communication and coordination. Teams may also find it useful to meet monthly or quarterly to discuss their work processes, troubleshoot problem areas, exchange program information and lessons learned, cross-train, and further build a sense of their identity as a team. Tasks should be delegated among team members in a way that allows for the most efficient care. For example, medical assistants or front desk staff may be trained to take on simple screenings or behavioral assessments, a role traditionally reserved for nursing and similar staff. Having providers from a range of disciplines work together as a team is more effective than usual care for chronic health conditions. Effective teams are characterized by their commitment to patient satisfaction, the presence of a team "champion," and a workable team size (neither too small nor too large) (Bodenheimer 2003).

MISSOURI CASE STUDY

The first SPA that was approved by CMS served eligible enrollees using CMHCs in Missouri. It was approved by CMS on October 20, 2011, and creates HHs in CMHCs for Medicaid enrollees with behavioral health conditions.

Program Design and Structure

The Missouri CMHC-HH program is overseen by the Medicaid authority, MO HealthNet, and is codirected by the Missouri Department of Mental Health. Other collaborating organizations include the Missouri Coalition of Community Mental Health Centers, Missouri Hospital Association, Missouri Foundation for Health, Health Care Foundation of Greater Kansas City, and Missouri Primary Care Association (representing FQHCs). The Department of Mental Health provides mental health services to the state of Missouri, particularly assisting those with SMI and children with severe emotional disturbances. The state's 29 CMHCs are the primary treatment providers for adults and children in child protective services, and all are part of the CMHC-HH program. They are also members of the Missouri Coalition of Community Mental Health Centers, a key collaborator on the CMHC-HH program, who also played a role in training and outreach to the member associations.

Missouri uses ProAct, an electronic health record and care management tool developed by Care Management Technologies, a provider of evidence-based behavioral health analytics and decision support tools. Care Management Technologies provides behavioral pharmacy, medication adherence, and disease management reports, which are key tools of the HH program as described in detail in the section "Missouri Definition: Six Health Home–Required Services." Several years prior to the HH project, Missouri implemented another all-provider Web-based electronic health record called CyberAccess, which allows providers to view claims-based diagnosis data and medication data, prescribe electronically, receive alerts, and request prior authorizations for Medicaid enrollees. CyberAccess is available to all Medicaid providers, including CMHC and primary care HH providers, and is used for care coordination and attestation in the HH program.

The CMHC-HH program was implemented at all 29 CMHCs in January 2012. Medicaid beneficiaries were enrolled in the CMHC-HH program through an autoenrollment process. Beneficiaries who were identified as meeting one of the three conditions outlined in the approved Missouri SPA and who met the Medicaid spending threshold of at least $10,000 were then autoenrolled and assigned to one of the designated HHs, as this particular population was deemed best able to achieve cost savings through better care coordination.

All of Missouri's 29 CMHCs serve as HHs, and each agreed to achieve HH certification from the Commission on Accreditation of Rehabilitation Facilities and to provide services to their assigned catchment area (25 total catchment areas for the state). The CMHC-HH philosophy and model of care involves provision of psychiatric rehabilitation services with a focus on facilitating disease management and care coordination, while also promoting independence and community integration. The goals of the HH are to improve access to services, promote healthy lifestyles, and educate enrollees on how to manage their own conditions and coordinate their care with other providers, including specialists, emergency departments, and hospitals.

Missouri Definition: Six Health Home-Required Services

1. *Comprehensive care management services* are conducted by the nurse care manager (NCM), PCP consultant, HH administrative support staff, and HH director, with the participation of other team members. It consists of identification of high-risk individuals and use of client information to determine level of participation in care management services; assessment of preliminary service needs; treatment plan development, which will include client goals, preferences, and optimal clinical outcomes; assignment of health team member roles and responsibilities; development of treatment guidelines that establish clinical pathways for health teams to follow across risk levels or health conditions; monitoring of individual and population health status and service use to determine adherence to or variance from treatment guidelines; and development and dissemination of reports that indicate progress toward meeting outcomes for client satisfaction, health status, service delivery, and costs.

2. *Care coordination* is the implementation of the individualized treatment plan (with active patient involvement) through appropriate linkages, referrals, coordination, and follow-up to needed services and supports, in-

cluding referral and linkages to long-term services and supports. Specific activities include, but are not limited to, the following: appointment scheduling, conducting referrals and follow-up monitoring, participating in hospital discharge processes, and communicating with other providers and clients/family members. NCMs, with the assistance of the HH administrative support staff, will be responsible for conducting care coordination activities across the health team. The primary responsibility of the NCM is to ensure implementation of the treatment plan for achievement of clinical outcomes consistent with the needs and preferences of the client.

3. *Health promotion services* shall minimally consist of providing health education specific to an individual's chronic conditions, development of self-management plans with the individual, education regarding the importance of immunizations and screenings, fostering child physical and emotional development, providing support for improving social networks, and providing health-promoting lifestyle interventions, including, but not limited to, substance use prevention, smoking prevention and cessation, nutritional counseling, obesity reduction and prevention, and increasing physical activity. Health promotion services also assist clients with participating in the implementation of their treatment plan and place a strong emphasis on person-centered empowerment to understand and self-manage chronic health conditions.

4. *Comprehensive transitional care* includes appropriate follow-up from inpatient to other settings. In conducting comprehensive transitional care, a member of the health team provides care coordination services designed to streamline plans of care, reduce hospital admissions, ease the transition to long-term services and supports, and interrupt patterns of frequent hospital emergency department use. The health team member collaborates with physicians, nurses, social workers, discharge planners, pharmacists, and others to continue implementation of the treatment plan, with a specific focus on increasing clients' and family members' ability to manage care and live safely in the community and shift the use of reactive care and treatment to proactive health promotion and self-management. The NCM and PCP consultant will participate in providing comprehensive transitional care activities, including, whenever possible, participating in discharge planning.

5. *Individual and family support services* activities include, but are not limited to, the following: advocating for individuals and families, assisting with obtaining and adhering to medications, and assisting with other prescribed treatments. In addition, health team members are responsible for identifying resources for individuals to support them in attaining their highest level of health and functioning in their families and in the com-

munity, including transportation to medically necessary services. A primary focus will be increasing health literacy and the ability to self-manage their care and facilitating participation in the ongoing revision of their care/treatment plan. For individuals with developmental disabilities, the health team will refer to and coordinate with the approved developmental disabilities case management entity for services more directly related to habilitation and coordinate with the approved developmental disabilities case management entity for services more directly related to a particular health care condition. NCMs will provide this service.

6. *Referral to community and social support services,* including long-term services and supports, involves providing assistance for clients to obtain and maintain eligibility for health care, disability benefits, housing, and personal need and legal services, as examples. For individuals with developmental disabilities, the health team will refer to and coordinate with the approved developmental disabilities case management entity for this service. The NCM and administrative support staff will provide this service.

Missouri Health Home Team

Each CMHC must have a HH director, NCM, PCP consultant, and care coordinators/community support workers (CSWs). The CMHC-HH payment model supports the following ratio of HH staff to patient enrollees:

- 1 HH director: 500 enrollees
- 1 NCM: 250 enrollees
- 1 hour of PCP consultant time per enrollee per year
- 1 care coordinator/CSW per 500 enrollees

Any additional staff employed by the HH must be funded outside the CMHC-HH payment model.

The role of the HH director is to oversee the practice transformation and training of the HH team. The NCMs ensure metabolic screening (lipid level, hemoglobin A1c, and blood pressure) is occurring at least annually for each enrollee in addition to helping patients develop health goals and care plans to manage their chronic health conditions. Annual metabolic screening is a required component of the CMHC-HH program and a key source of clinical data for care management. NCMs review the claims-based diagnosis, medication, medication adherence, and treatment history reports generated by the Care Management Technologies care management tool ProAct and coordinate follow-up with enrollees if they have been discharged from a hospital. NCMs may organize health fairs and conduct classes on topics such as tobacco cessation to raise awareness among HH enrollees, staff, and the broader CMHC-HH membership.

The PCP consultant is one of the more prominent additions to the CMHCs as a result of the HH program funding. The consultant does not provide any direct care to the enrollee, unless he or she happens to be the enrollee's primary care physician outside the CMHC. The physician consultant's role is to assist the CMHCs in strengthening their primary care coordination activities. The duties of the Missouri PCP consultants are listed in the section "Health Home Team." Some examples of their work many include an "ask the doc" session for patients, which allows them to better understand their diagnosis and medication regimens. Brown bag lunches for staff help educate them about chronic health conditions so they can better explain and track these in their patients. The PCP consultant provides a unique opportunity to partner with the in-house psychiatric team to review patients with chronic conditions, consult on urgent issues, and retrain them in the current treatment of common conditions. PCP consultants write letters to their outside specialist or primary care physician with suggestions for altering their medication or care plan. These letters are not always well received, and may be ignored, by outside physicians, while at other times they are appreciated, thus highlighting the PCP consultant's important role in fostering positive relationships with these providers.

Primary Care Provider Consultant Role in the Missouri Health Home

The health care home has very much become part of the culture now. It is fascinating to attempt to apply baseline medical care on a population-based scale. Mainly, I believe our clients benefit from our efforts, which is the way I measure the success of the program.

J.G., PCP consultant, Missouri

The CSW is the HH team member with the most direct and frequent contact with the HH enrollees. The CSW role is not new to CMHCs, as CSWs were also part of the Department of Mental Health's preexisting Comprehensive Psychiatric Rehabilitation program. However, as a result of the HH program, CSWs are now better trained to help enrollees manage their health conditions. The CSWs work with the enrollees to complete the day-to-day tasks related to maintaining their health. This might include helping them make appointments for other medical care, schedule transportation to appointments, pick up prescriptions, purchase healthy foods, or maintain a fitness plan. CSWs often attend appointments with enrollees to make sure that the primary care physician consultants' suggestions are shared with the enrollees' other health care providers. CSWs are provided training by PCP consultants and NCMs in chronic medical illness and wellness lifestyle to facilitate their new role as wellness coaches.

Payment in the Missouri Health Home

The CMHC-HH receives a $78.74 PMPM fee to cover the cost of a HH director, NCM, PCP consultant, and care coordinators/case managers. In order to receive payments, HH sites must attest monthly to providing HH services required by Section 2703. At a minimum, this includes providing monitoring for HH enrollees for health care gaps that require care coordination or disease management intervention and keeping records of the monitoring for auditing purposes. Examples of services that meet the criteria for payment include phone calls to the enrollee to discuss care plans, follow-up after hospital discharges, and face-to-face meetings with an NCM, CSW, or PCP consultant. Payments are given only for those patients who are Medicaid-eligible and meet the spend-down criteria (documentation of medical care expenses that cover the amount that is in excess of the limit to qualify for Medicaid) by the last day of the month. The funding provided to the CMHC provider organizations through the CMHC-HH program did not supplant any previous funding they received prior to becoming a HH.

Results of the Missouri Health Home Implementation

Since implementation of the per patient per month payments, HHs have provided the vast majority of enrollees with broad access to needed medications; improved performance on various processes, including metabolic screening (increase from 12% to 61%) and postdischarge follow-up; improved chronic disease outcome measures, including improved diabetes, hypertension, and lipid measures; and reduced utilization and costs (12.8% decline in hospital admissions, 8.2% drop in emergency room visits) (Department of Mental Health and MO HealthNet 2013).

CONCLUSION

The PPACA, Section 2703, which authorizes health homes for persons with chronic conditions, offers psychiatrists and the CMHCs they work in an opportunity to simultaneously reduce the excess morbidity and premature mortality of their patients, integrate with primary care providers, and build a new role for themselves in the larger health care system by providing coordinated medical oversight for the sickest, most complicated, and most expensive patients. Missouri's implementation of Section 2703 has proven effective in improving health care outcomes and reducing the total cost of care.

REFERENCES

Agency for Healthcare Research and Quality: Defining the PCMH. Rockville, MD, Agency for Healthcare Research and Quality, 2013. Available at: http://pcmh.ahrq.gov/page/defining-pcmh. Accessed December 6, 2013.

AIMS Center: Patient-Centered Integrated Behavioral Health Care Principles and Tasks. Seattle, WA, AIMS Center, 2011. Available at: http://uwaims.org/overview-principles.html. Accessed December 6, 2013.

Alakeson V, Frank RG, Katz RE: Specialty care medical homes for people with severe, persistent mental disorders. Health Aff (Millwood) 29(5):867–873, 2010

American Academy of Family Physicians, American Academy of Pediatrics, American College of Physicians, et al: Joint principles of the patient-centered medical home. Washington, DC, Patient-Centered Primary Care Collaborative, February 2007. Available at: http://www.aafp.org/dam/AAFP/documents/practice_management/pcmh/initiatives/PCMHJoint.pdf. Accessed May 24, 2014.

Bodenheimer T: Interventions to improve chronic illness care: evaluating their effectiveness. Dis Manag 6(2):63–71, 2003

Bodenheimer T, Berry-Millet R: The Synthesis Project: Care Management of Patients With Complex Health Care Needs. Princeton, NJ, Robert Wood Johnson Foundation, 2009. Available at: http://www.rwjf.org/content/dam/farm/reports/issue_briefs/2009/rwjf49853/subassets/rwjf49853_1. Accessed December 6, 2013.

Colton CW, Manderscheid RW: Congruencies in increased mortality rates, years of potential life lost, and causes of death among public mental health clients in eight states. Prev Chronic Dis 3(2):1–14, 2006

Council on Pediatric Practice: Standards of Child Health Care. Evanston, IL, American Academy of Pediatrics, 1967

Department of Mental Health and MO HealthNet: Progress report: Missouri CMHC healthcare homes. November 2013. Available at dmh.mo.gov/docs/mentalillness/18MonthReport.pdf. Accessed May 24, 2014.

Druss BG, von Esenwein SA: Improving general medical care for persons with mental and addictive disorders: systematic review. Gen Hosp Psychiatry 28(2):145–153, 2006

Druss BG, Walker ER: The Synthesis Project: Mental Disorders and Medical Comorbidity. Research Synthesis Report No 21. Princeton, NJ, Robert Wood Johnson Foundation, 2011. Available at: http://www.mdhelpsd.org/downloads/medicalcomorbidity.pdf. Accessed December 6, 2013.

Druss BG, von Esenwein SA, Compton MT, et al: A randomized trial of medical care management for community mental health settings: the Primary Care Access, Referral, and Evaluation (PCARE) study. Am J Psychiatry 167(2):151–159, 2010a

Druss BG, Zhao L, von Esenwein SA, et al: The Health and Recovery Peer (HARP) Program: a peer-led intervention to improve medical self-management for persons with serious mental illness. Schizophr Res 118(1–3):264–270, 2010b

Goodwin K, Tobler L: Community Health Workers Expanding the Scope of the Health Care Delivery System. Washington, DC, National Council of State Legislatures, 2008. Available at: http://www.ncsl.org/print/health/CHWBrief.pdf. Accessed December 6, 2013.

Halpern R, Boulter P: Population-Based Health Care: Definitions and Applications. Boston, MA, Tufts Health Care Institute, November 2000.

Mann C: Re: Health Homes for Enrollees With Chronic Conditions (letter to state Medicaid directors and state health officials) SMDL# 10–024 ACA# 12. Baltimore, MD, Center for Medicaid and CHIP Services, November 16, 2010. Available at: http://downloads.cms.gov/cmsgov/archived-downloads/SMDL/downloads/SMD10024.pdf. Accessed December 6, 2013.

Mann C: Re: Integrated Care Models (letter to state Medicaid director) SMDL# 12–001 ICM# 1. Baltimore, MD, Center for Medicaid and CHIP Services, July 10, 2012. Available at: http://www.medicaid.gov/Federal-Policy-Guidance/downloads/SMD-12-001.pdf. Accessed December 6, 2013.

Parks J, Pollack D, Bartels S, et al: Integrating Behavioral Health and Primary Care Services: Opportunities and Challenges for State Mental Health Authorities. 11th Technical Report. Alexandria, VA, National Association of State Mental Health Program Directors Medical Directors Council, January 2005. Available at: http://www.nasmhpd.org/docs/publications/MDCdocs/Final%20Technical%20Report%20on%20Primary%20Care%20-%20Behavioral%20Health%20Integration.final.pdf. Accessed December 6, 2013.

Parks J, Svendsen D, Singer P, et al: Morbidity and Mortality in People With Serious Mental Illness. 13th Technical Report. Alexandria, VA, National Association of State Mental Health Program Directors Medical Directors Council, October 2006. Available at: http://www.dsamh.utah.gov/docs/mortality-morbidity_nasmhpd.pdf. Accessed December 6, 2013.

Parks J, Radke AQ, Mazade NA, et al: Measurement of Health Status for People With Serious Mental Illnesses. 16th Technical Report. Alexandria, VA, National Association of State Mental Health Program Directors Medical Directors Council, October 16, 2008. Available at: http://www.nasmhpd.org/docs/publications/MDCdocs/NASMHPD%20Medical%20Directors%20Health%20Indicators%20Report%2011-19-08.pdf. Accessed December 6, 2013.

Parks J, Johnson M, Raney L, et al: Primary care provider consultant role in the Missouri health home. Panel discussion at Healthcare Home Physician Institute Summit, Missouri Department of Mental Health, Branson, MO, June 12, 2012

Parks J, Johnson M, Raney L, et al: Psychiatric provider role in the Missouri health home. Panel discussion at Healthcare Home Physician Institute Summit, Missouri Department of Mental Health, St. Charles, MO, October 2013

Salzer MS, Schwenk E, Brusilovskiy E: Certified peer specialist roles and activities: results from a national survey. Psychiatr Serv 61(5):520–523, 2010

Substance Abuse and Mental Health Services Administration: Promoting Recovery in Health Homes. Rockville, MD, Substance Abuse and Mental Health Services Administration, 2014

World Health Organization: WHO Disability Assessment Schedule 2.0. Geneva, Switzerland, World Health Organization, 2012. Available at: http://www.who.int/classifications/icf/whodasii/en/. Accessed December 6, 2013.

CHAPTER 10

Management of Leading Risk Factors for Cardiovascular Disease

Erik R. Vanderlip, M.D., M.P.H.

Lydia Chwastiak, M.D., M.P.H.

In this chapter, we intend to provide mental health practitioners with updated, evidence-based guidelines in the management of the most common modifiable risk factors for cardiovascular disease (CVD) (obesity, diabetes, dyslipidemia, hypertension, tobacco use disorders), the leading cause of mortality for adults with severe and persistent mental illness (Colton and Manderscheid 2006; Crump et al. 2013a, 2013b). The following sections provide a framework for screening, care management, and therapeutic risk reduction in this vulnerable population. By focusing on pragmatic approaches that may be pursued within the psychiatric scope of practice, we aim to equip psychiatrists with the tools necessary to understand and work within an integrated primary care system. A single case will be used to highlight various clinical points over the course of the chapter in each of the sections and will be referred to at various points throughout the chapter.

Case Example: Chapter-Wide Illustrative Case

B.H. is a 46-year-old white male with a history of chronic schizophrenia. You've known B.H. for about 10 years. When he first came to see you, he had just been discharged from his sixth hospitalization in his lifetime and had been placed on a long-acting injectable form of risperidone. This, in addition to intensive case management and supportive housing, has helped him dramatically reduce his reliance on in-hospital care and live more independently. The two times in the past 10 years that he has required hospitalizations have been when he was relatively nonadherent to his oral antipsychotic and became gravely disorganized. During one of these episodes, he was found outside his apartment by the police and needed to be admitted for hypothermia; he lost two toes on his right foot to frostbite. After the last hospitalization, about 18 months ago, he was switched to olanzapine (in addition to his long-acting injectable), and currently he has manageable symptoms when adherent to 20 mg/day.

B.H. has a payee to assist in managing his finances, though it remains a contentious issue. He tends to spend his extra money on canned foods, cola drinks/energy drinks, tobacco (he rolls his own cigarettes), and marijuana, and he often missed rent payments prior to the assignment of his payee. He lives in a supported housing development near the mental health clinic. Lately, you've been seeing B.H. about once a month; he usually rides the bus or takes a cab to the clinic with a voucher. There's a fast-food chain by your clinic where he sometimes eats meals. He looks heavier over the past year, though you think he was overweight even when you first saw him.

B.H.'s priorities are ever-increasing financial independence and, potentially, engaging in a meaningful romantic relationship.

OBESITY

Case Presentation

When you see B.H. in clinic today, you measure his weight. He weighs 287 lbs. You decide to try to calculate his body mass index (BMI). Because B.H. is a little taller than you, you estimate his height at 6'1" and perform an Internet search for an online BMI calculator. After plugging in the numbers, you discover B.H.'s BMI is 37.9. Looking back through his records, you have a weight from 2 years ago before the olanzapine, when he weighed 210 lbs (BMI 27.7). You wonder:

- Just how bad is his BMI?
- What can I do to help B.H. with his weight?

Background and Significance

Obesity is a leading cause of preventable death in the United States, second only to smoking (www.cdc.gov/obesity/data/adult.html). There is an epidemic of obesity in the United States, with devastating consequences among persons with serious mental illness (SMI), and more than half of individuals with SMI treated in public mental health clinics are obese (Correll et al. 2010).

Obesity is typically defined by BMI, a direct calculation based on height and weight. Generally, a BMI of 25 or more indicates that an individual is overweight, and 30 or more classifies the individual as obese (National

Heart, Lung and Blood Institute 1998). Waist circumference (measuring abdominal or central adiposity), which is highly correlated with insulin resistance, is emerging as a valid and reliable predictor of risk for type 2 diabetes and CVD (Correll and Frederickson 2006).

Metabolic syndrome describes a constellation of risk factors that confer a fivefold to sixfold increased risk of developing type 2 diabetes and threefold to sixfold increased risk of mortality due to CVD (Alberti et al. 2009) (Table 10–1). Metabolic syndrome is highly prevalent among patients with schizophrenia and bipolar disorder, with rates of 22%–30% or higher (Fagiolini et al. 2005; McEvoy et al. 2005).

TABLE 10–1. Criteria for metabolic syndrome (three or more of the following)

Criterion	NCEP ATP III, IDF, and AHA/NHLBI
Obesity	Waist circumference ≥ 102 cm in men and ≥ 88 cm in women
Triglyceride level	≥ 150 mg/dL
HDL cholesterol	< 40 mg/dL in men; < 50 mg/dL in women
Blood pressure	≥ 130/85 mm Hg or treatment with antihypertensive medication
Glucose	≥ 100 mg/dL

Note.   AHA = American Heart Association; HDL = high-density lipoprotein; IDF = International Diabetes Foundation; NCEP ATP III = National Cholesterol Education Program Adult Treatment Panel III; NHLBI = National Heart, Lung and Blood Institute.
Source.   Adapted from Expert Panel on Detection, Evaluation, and Treatment of High Blood Cholesterol in Adults 2001.

Screening and Diagnosis of Obesity and Metabolic Syndrome

Given the relationship between second-generation antipsychotic medications and the development of cardiovascular risk factors, in 2004 the American Diabetes Association and American Psychiatric Association recommended regular monitoring to identify and rapidly address medication-induced cardiometabolic side effects, including 1) consideration of metabolic risks when starting a second-generation antipsychotic medication; 2) patient and family education; 3) baseline screening of BMI, blood pressure (BP), waist circumference, fasting glucose, and a fasting lipid profile; 4) regular monitoring of these cardiovascular risk factors; and 5) referral to specialized services to decrease risk (American Diabetes Association et al. 2004; Table 10–2). Adoption of these recommendations has been slow, and evidence-based interventions to promote weight loss or decrease diabetes risk are not typically available at most community mental health centers.

Psychiatrists should (regardless of medications prescribed) monitor and chart weight and BMI at every visit and should encourage patients to monitor their own weight.

TABLE 10–2. Recommendations for metabolic monitoring of patients treated with second-generation antipsychotic medications

	Baseline	4 Weeks	8 Weeks	12 Weeks	Every 3 months	Annually
Personal or family history of obesity, dyslipidemia, hypertension, diabetes, or CVD	X					X
Weight (BMI)	X	X	X	X	X	
Waist circumference	X					X
Blood pressure	X			X		X
Fasting glucose	X			X		X
Fasting lipids	X			X		X

Note. BMI = body mass index; CVD = cardiovascular disease.
Source. Copyright 2004 American Diabetes Association. From *Diabetes Care*, Vol. 27, 2004; 596–601. Modified with permission from The American Diabetes Association.

Treatment of Obesity

Lifestyle Modification

Weight loss through a healthy lifestyle (increased physical activity and decreased caloric intake) can prevent or delay the onset of type 2 diabetes and CVD, particularly in high-risk individuals. Even small reductions in body weight can lead to substantial improvements in a metabolic risk profile: weight loss of as little as 5% of initial body weight can postpone the onset of or prevent type 2 diabetes, hypertension, hyperlipidemia, and CVD (Goldstein 1992) (Table 10–3). Insulin sensitivity improves rapidly before much weight loss occurs and continues to improve with continued weight loss (Knowler et al. 2002).

Manualized lifestyle interventions, such as the Diabetes Prevention Program, have substantial evidence of effectiveness in promoting weight loss (Ali et al. 2012). Such interventions have been adapted to address psychiatric symptoms and neurocognitive impairment, and several large randomized controlled trials have demonstrated the efficacy of lifestyle interventions among persons with SMI (Bonfioli et al. 2012; Daumit et al. 2013).

TABLE 10–3. Beneficial effects of leading cardiovascular risk factor interventions

Risk factor	Change	Associated risk reduction
Blood cholesterol	↓10% total cholesterol[a]	30% CVD
Blood pressure	↓6 mm Hg[b]	16% CVD 42% stroke
Diabetes	↓HbA1c 1%[c]	21% type 2 diabetes–related deaths 14% myocardial infarction 37% microvascular complications
Tobacco use	Cessation[d]	50% CVD
Obesity	Maintenance of normal body weight *or* loss of 5%–10% body weight[e]	35%–55% CVD
Increased physical activity	30-minute daily walk[f]	35%–55% CVD

Note. CVD=cardiovascular disease.
Source. [a]Stone et al. 2013; [b]Chobanian et al. 2003; [c]Stratton et al. 2000; [d]Critchley and Capewell 2003; [e]Goldstein 1992; [f]Chiuve et al. 2011.

Patients (and their families) should be educated about healthy lifestyles. This education does not need to be administered by a nutritionist or other specialist; it can be administered effectively by mental health clinic staff. Psychiatrists, nurses, and other members of the mental health team can educate and motivate patients with SMI to make lifestyle modifications with respect to diet and exercise.

Emerging models of peer-supported community mental health interventions specifically addressing obesity and health are available through the Substance Abuse and Mental Health Services Administration's Center for Integrated Health Solutions (www.integration.samhsa.gov). Specific interventions include Whole Health Action Management and the Health and Recovery Peer Program—both of which offer consumer-oriented solutions to managing health and recovery.

Pharmacotherapy for Obesity

Before consideration of additional medications to treat obesity, thought should be given to switching from an antipsychotic medication with a higher weight-gain liability to one with a lower weight-gain liability, as discussed in Chapter 7 ("The Case for Primary Care in Public Mental Health Settings"). Pharmacologic treatments can reduce weight gain induced by antipsychotic medication in some patients. To date, most evidence exists for metformin

(500–1,000 mg twice daily) and topiramate (50–200 mg daily in divided doses) (Correll et al. 2010; Jarskog et al. 2013; Maayan et al. 2010). Treatment with these medications should be reserved for individuals who have gained a significant amount of weight on an antipsychotic (more than 7% from baseline) that cannot be safely replaced by a less metabolically active compound and for persons unable to make significant diet and lifestyle modifications. There is no clear expert consensus on when to start these medications outside of specific indications (diabetes) or for how long to treat, and patients should be counseled on their rationale for use and potential risks and benefits prior to the initiation of therapy. Numerous weight loss drugs have recently emerged on the market, but none have been proven safe or effective for those with SMI. Their use should be entertained only after informed discussion with patients and careful evaluation of alternative, proven therapies.

Bariatric Surgery

Bariatric surgery is indicated for patients who do not succeed with nonsurgical intervention and who have class III obesity (BMI of 40 or greater) or medically complicated class II obesity (BMI of 35–39.9 or greater). Long-term studies show the procedures cause significant loss of weight, recovery from diabetes, improvement in cardiovascular risk factors, and a 23% reduction in mortality (Kashyap et al. 2013; Vest et al. 2013). In 2011, the International Diabetes Federation Taskforce on Epidemiology and Prevention of Diabetes recommended bariatric surgery as an appropriate treatment for people with type 2 diabetes and obesity who have been unable to achieve recommended treatment targets using medical therapies, particularly if other major comorbidities exist (Dixon et al. 2011). There are limited data about the efficacy and tolerability of bariatric surgery among patients with SMI, but some preliminary results support outcomes comparable to those for individuals without SMI (Ahmed et al. 2013; Hamoui et al. 2004).

Case Discussion

After talking with B.H., you review his chart and discuss switching from olanzapine to aripiprazole, because he's never been on that before. Both of you are reluctant to make the change now, because he is tolerating the olanzapine well. You both opt to have him start walking to your clinical appointments and to transition to only diet soda consumption. You offer a referral to primary care but acknowledge that B.H. doesn't like medical clinics. He's technically enrolled in the local primary care clinic several blocks up the street, but he has not been there for over 3 years, and you don't know any of their providers since they seem to change frequently. You decide to go ahead and check some lab values, including his blood sugar, because you think he is at risk for developing diabetes.

Clinical Pearls: Obesity

- Start with small, manageable goals in diet and lifestyle changes that can easily be attained and sustained over time.
- Advocate for exercise. It can take all forms, and small amounts of physical activity can lead to greater amounts over time. Working walking or taking the stairs into daily routines can be a great place to start.
- Consider switching antipsychotic therapy to less metabolically active compounds in patients who are symptom-stable.

DIABETES

Case Presentation

You order some labs for B.H. from your clinic. They include blood glucose, lipid profile, serum electrolytes, liver function, and complete blood count. They return when you are in the office a week later. You realize that B.H. wasn't fasting when he had his blood work done because it was in the afternoon. His blood sugar is 195 mg/dL. After calling B.H. to discuss the labs, you put in an order for a hemoglobin A1c, and it returns at 6.1%. You wonder:

- Does B.H. have diabetes?
- What can be done to help B.H. avoid further medical complications in the future?

Background and Significance

More than 25 million people in the United States have type 2 diabetes (8.3% of the population), and diabetes was the seventh leading cause of death in 2011 (www.cdc.gov/diabetes/pubs/pdf/ndfs_2011.pdf). Almost 20% of Medicaid enrollees with diabetes have a co-occurring mental illness (Druss et al. 2012), and among patients with diabetes, the presence of psychiatric illness is associated with increased rates of diabetes complications, diabetes-related hospitalizations, and diabetes-specific mortality (Becker and Hux 2011; Mai et al. 2011). Chapter 7 reviews the association of some psychotropic medications and diabetes and relationships between SMI and diabetes outcomes. A comprehensive discussion of the following management recommendations is provided by the American Diabetes Association (2013) in an annual report.

Type 2 diabetes is a disorder of metabolism characterized by hyperglycemia, resulting from either inadequate insulin secretion or resistance to insulin action. Type 1 diabetes is an autoimmune disorder that results from beta-cell destruction, leading to insulin deficiency. The vast majority

(90%–95%) of patients with diabetes have type 2 diabetes (http://diabetes.niddk.nih.gov/dm/pubs/overview/). In patients with type 2 diabetes, insulin is produced, but it is ineffective in target tissues, and there is an inadequate secretory response to nutrient intake. The clinical presence of type 2 diabetes is usually the culmination of years of metabolic stress that begins well before laboratory markers indicate hyperglycemia, with most individuals eventually progressing toward insulin dependence. Other forms of diabetes also exist, the most common being gestational-onset. Complications of diabetes are divided primarily into microvascular (e.g., retinal, renal, neuropathic disease) and macrovascular (e.g., coronary artery, cerebrovascular, peripheral vascular disease).

The use and availability of the percentage of glycosylated hemoglobin (hemoglobin A1c, HbA1c, "A1c") as a screening test and treatment monitor have expanded greatly in the past decade. HbA1c is formed by hemoglobin's exposure to plasma glucose and reflects the average plasma glucose concentration over a 2- to 3-month period of time. It can vary depending on the relative turnover of hemoglobin, such that those with higher turnover (e.g., recent anemia, blood transfusions) may have artificially low HbA1c levels.

Screening and Diagnosis of Diabetes

Annual screening for type 2 diabetes in asymptomatic people should be considered in adults of any age who are overweight or obese (BMI 25 or greater) and those who have one or more risk factors for diabetes, including treatment with a second-generation antipsychotic medication (American Diabetes Association et al. 2004). Adults with a history of prediabetes or gestational-onset diabetes are also candidates for yearly screening, while adults with hypertension or metabolic syndrome should be screened every other year. Adults at average risk should be screened every 3 years beginning at age 45.

Table 10–4 summarizes the recommendations for diagnosis of diabetes. In 2010, the American Diabetes Association adopted the HbA1c threshold of ≥6.5% as diagnostic of diabetes (American Diabetes Association 2010). Prediabetes is based on impaired fasting glucose (100–125 mg/dL), impaired glucose tolerance (2-hour values of oral glucose-tolerance test of 140–199 mg/dL), or HbA1c (5.7%–6.4%). Individuals with an HbA1c of 6.0%–6.5% have a significantly elevated risk of progressing to full-blown diabetes.

The HbA1c test is less sensitive than fasting glucose level as a diagnostic screen. This lower sensitivity may well be offset by the test's greater practicality, however, because it does not require fasting or timed samples. Point-of-care HbA1c assays (finger-stick machines) are now widely available and may increase the feasibility of screening for diabetes at community mental

TABLE 10–4. American Diabetes Association recommendations for diagnosing diabetes

Test	Results	Interpretation
A1c	<5.7%	Normal
	5.7%–6.4%	Prediabetes
	6.5% or higher on two separate days	Diabetes
Fasting plasma glucose	<100 mg/dL	Normal
	100–125 mg/dL	Prediabetes (impaired fasting glucose)
	126 mg/dL or higher on two separate days	Diabetes
Random plasma glucose	<140 mg/dL	Normal
	140–199 mg/dL	Prediabetes
	200 mg/dL or higher on two separate days	Diabetes

Source. International Expert Committee: "International Expert Committee Report on the Role of the A1c Assay in the Diagnosis of Diabetes." *Diabetes Care* 32(7):1327–1334, 2009.

health centers. Their use for diagnostic purposes could be problematic, so a blood test is still recommended (American Diabetes Association 2013). A test result diagnostic of diabetes should be repeated to rule out laboratory error.

Treatment of Prediabetes and Diabetes

Prediabetes

Individuals with prediabetes should be informed of their increased risk for diabetes and CVD (American Diabetes Association 2013). Follow-up should be particularly vigilant (at minimum every 6 months) for those with HbA1c above 6.0%. Some data indicate interventions targeted at individuals with prediabetes may have the greatest overall return on health for the population. Patients with prediabetes should be referred to an effective ongoing support program, such as the Diabetes Prevention Program (http://diabetes.niddk.nih.gov/dm/pubs/preventionprogram/). Such structured programs that emphasize lifestyle changes of moderate weight loss (5%–10% of body weight), regular physical activity (150 minutes per week), and dietary strategies of reduced calories and reduced intake of dietary fat can reduce the risk of developing diabetes (Knowler et al. 2002). Several large randomized controlled trials have demonstrated the efficacy of lifestyle modification programs among patients with SMI (Bonfioli et al. 2012; Daumit et al. 2013; Wu et al. 2008). To date, such programs have not been widely implemented in community mental health centers.

The use of medication such as metformin has some potential in preventing the progression from prediabetes to diabetes but has not reached standard of care and may not be as successful as intensive lifestyle modification (Goldberg et al. 2009).

Diabetes

At the time of diagnosis, management of hyperglycemia in most patients with type 2 diabetes should begin with lifestyle modification. The goals in caring for patients with diabetes mellitus are to eliminate symptoms and to prevent or delay the development of complications. Diabetes care requires multifactorial risk reduction strategies beyond glycemic control. This includes microvascular risk reduction through control of hyperglycemia and BP and macrovascular risk reduction through control of lipids and hypertension, smoking cessation, and aspirin therapy.

A complete medical evaluation should be performed to detect the presence of complications, review previous treatment and risk factor control, and assist in formulating a management plan. All treatment decisions should involve the patient, with a focus on preferences, needs, and values. Psychosocial assessment should include attitudes about the illness, expectation about medical management and outcomes, mood, quality of life, social support, and psychiatric history.

Self-Management

Support and education with respect to diabetes self-management is a critical component of diabetes care. Self-management includes setting appropriate goals, lifestyle modification (described in section "Diet and Lifestyle Modification"), foot care, and in some patients medications and glucose self-monitoring. Glucose self-monitoring is useful only if patients are testing and are using the information to make changes in their treatment regimen (insulin or insulin secretagogues). Patients using multiple insulin injections should monitor glucose at least 3 times a day. It is not typically necessary for patients on lifestyle modification or metformin alone to monitor finger-stick glucoses, because they are not at risk for hypoglycemia.

Diet and Lifestyle Modification

Diet and exercise are the foundation of diabetes treatment. Caloric restriction is of primary importance. After that, individuals may exercise their preferences for types of dietary intake. Providers should advocate a diet composed of foods that are within the financial reach and cultural milieu of the patient. Limiting intake of sugar-sweetened beverages, simple sugars, and saturated fats while achieving the recommended dietary fiber intake (14 g fiber/1,000 kcal) is a relatively simple initial recommendation. For personalized eating plans and interactive tools to help patients evaluate food choices, see the U.S. Department of Agriculture's Choose My Plate Web site (www.choosemyplate.gov).

Adults with type 2 diabetes should be advised to perform at least 150 minutes per week of moderate-intensity aerobic physical activity (50%–70% of maximum heart rate, which is approximated by subtracting age from 220) spread over at least 3 days per week, with no more than 2 consecutive days without exercise. For patients who have been inactive, slowly working up to at least 30 minutes of moderate physical activity per day is acceptable, and this activity may be divided into 10- to 15-minute sessions throughout the day. When possible, patients should choose an activity they are likely to continue. Older patients, patients with long-standing disease, patients with multiple risk factors, and patients with previous evidence of atherosclerotic disease should have a cardiovascular evaluation prior to beginning a significant exercise regimen.

Pharmacologic Treatment

For individuals with an initial HbA1c between 6.5% and 7.5%, monotherapy with metformin is the preferred agent (Nathan et al. 2009). Metformin decreases the risk of mortality when used to treat type 2 diabetes and should be a standard part of combination treatments unless it is contraindicated. Patients with serum creatinine above 1.5 mg/dL, congestive heart failure, or age greater than 80 years are at increased risk of lactic acidosis and should not take metformin. Advantages of metformin include low level of side effects (in particular, weight gain), relatively low cost, and absence of hypoglycemia. The dose of metformin is titrated over 1–2 months up to 2,000 mg/day, administered in divided doses (during or after meals to reduce gastrointestinal side effects).

Individuals with an HbA1c between 7.6% and 9% usually require combination drug therapy. If the patient does not safely achieve or sustain glycemic goals within 2–3 months, either a sulfonylurea or basal insulin should be added (Table 10–5). Failure of initial therapy usually results in addition of another class of drug rather than substitution. Substitution should be reserved for cases in which patients experience intolerance to a drug because of adverse effects.

Individuals with an initial HbA1c greater than 9% will likely require insulin therapy to achieve glycemic targets. Owing to the progressive nature of type 2 diabetes, insulin therapy is eventually indicated for many patients. Insulin therapy is initiated based on a weekly average of blood sugars. The patient should be instructed to check fasting blood sugar every day, and insulin can be initiated and titrated to a target mean fasting (morning and before meals) blood sugar of 120 mg/dL.

TABLE 10–5.   Pharmacotherapy for type 2 diabetes

Class	Drug and dosing	Side effects	Contraindications	Notes
Biguanides	Metformin (500–1,000 mg twice daily, no benefit above 2,000 mg/day)	GI symptoms (diarrhea/loose stools, nausea, usually improved after 1 week) Metallic taste	Renal insufficiency (Cr > 1.5 mg/dL contraindicated, higher risk of lactic acidosis) Imaging study with IV contrast	Should be mainstay of treatment, no hypoglycemia (euglycemic), associated with modest weight loss
Sulfonylureas	Glipizide (2.5–40 mg/day, divided twice daily above 15 mg daily) Glyburide (1.25–20 mg/day)	Hypoglycemia, weight gain	Previous intolerance, sulfa allergy	Extended-release forms available, but widely available as generic
Thiazolidinediones (TZDs, glitazones)	Rosiglitazone (4–8 mg once daily) Pioglitazone (15–45 mg/day)	Anemia, swelling (edema), fluid retention, weight gain, bone loss and osteoporotic fractures in women	Congestive heart failure, history of myocardial infarction, liver disease (requires LFT monitoring)	Third-line agent only to be used when metformin and SUs have been exhausted and insulin is not an option
GLP-1 analogue	Exenatide (Byetta) (5–10 mcg sq twice daily)	Nausea, headache, hypoglycemia (when used with SUs), rarely pancreatitis	Affordability, sq injection	Expensive and less desirable than basal and bolus insulin, may promote weight loss

TABLE 10–5. Pharmacotherapy for type 2 diabetes *(continued)*

Class	Drug and dosing	Side effects	Contraindications	Notes
Basal insulin	Insulin glargine (Lantus) Starting dose in insulin-naïve patients: 10 U sq once daily (or 0.2 U/kg)	Hypoglycemia, weight gain, injection site reaction	No absolute contraindications	Should have specific education from clinical team instructing on use, what to do in event of hypoglycemic emergency, can be taken anytime during the day, needs to be consistent, available in convenient SoloSTAR delivery system, many Medicaid plans will cover

Note. Cr=creatinine; GI=gastrointestinal; GLP-1=glucagon-like peptide–1; IV=intravenous; LFT=liver function test; sq=subcutaneous; SUs=sulfonylureas; U=unit.

Treat to Target

Chronic hyperglycemia is associated with an increased risk of microvascular complications (Diabetes Control and Complications Trial/Epidemiology of Diabetes Interventions and Complications (DCCT/EDIC) Study Research Group 2005; UK Prospective Diabetes Study [UKPDS] Group 1998). Overall, studies suggest that tight glycemic control (HbA1c 7% or lower) is valuable for microvascular and macrovascular disease risk reduction only in patients with recent-onset disease, no known CVDs, and a longer life expectancy.

Glycemic targets and glucose-lowering therapies should be individualized. In patients with known CVD, advanced microvascular or macrovascular complications or complex comorbidity, longer duration of diabetes (15 or more years), and a shorter life expectancy, tighter glycemic control is not as beneficial (particularly with regard to CVD risk). Episodes of severe hypoglycemia may be particularly harmful in older individuals with existing CVD. A less stringent goal (less than 8%) may be appropriate for these patients—or for any patient above 60 years of age.

Recommendations for monitoring patients with diabetes are summarized in the American Diabetes Association annual reports. Generally, individuals with diabetes should be screened yearly for nephropathy with urine microalbumin, retinopathy with dilated eye exams, and neuropathy with foot exams and monofilament testing (while also checking for signs of skin breakdown or ulcer formation). Treatment of diabetes should include specific efforts at comprehensive reduction of cardiovascular risk, including smoking cessation, BP control, statin therapy for dyslipidemia, use of an angiotensin converting enzyme (ACE) inhibitor or an angiotensin II receptor blocker (ARB) to target microalbuminuria, and antiplatelet therapy (aspirin). First-line treatment for patients with diabetes and hypertension is an ACE inhibitor or an ARB. Additionally, there is mounting evidence on the effectiveness of bariatric surgery in reducing diabetes, and it should be considered in the context of refractory obesity as noted earlier in the section "Bariatric Surgery."

The wide availability of HbA1c measures allows for relatively easy management of type 2 diabetes. When possible, the utilization of a disease registry to list, track, and manage diabetic or prediabetic patients over time is recommended. Clinical processes should ensure HbA1c monitoring ideally every 3 months, with aggressive diet, lifestyle, and pharmacotherapy management to ensure that HbA1c reductions are met (see section "Pharmacologic Treatment") and clients not engaged in care are proactively identified to ensure proper follow-up.

Case Discussion

B.H. is at particularly high risk for developing diabetes, though technically he falls into the prediabetes range. There are a number of highly effective interventions, which can include intensive diet/lifestyle modifications, that may help B.H. fight off the onset of diabetes in the short run, and a referral to a local self-management group may help too. At this point, there is also evidence to support the use of metformin or, perhaps, topiramate to help him with weight loss. Prior to that, however, considerable thought should now be given to switching B.H. to a less metabolically active antipsychotic, such as aripiprazole, ziprasidone, or perphenazine. Additionally, there is mounting evidence that B.H. is having medical complications with his obesity, and weight loss surgery could even be considered, though clearly intensive diet and lifestyle modifications would be associated with lower risk.

The next time you see B.H., you discuss his lab results and his prediabetes and decide that in addition to his walking and switch to diet soda, you're going to try aripiprazole and have him come back in a month for follow-up. You remind yourself to review his weight, BP, and HbA1c 1–3 months into treatment on aripiprazole in addition to his psychiatric symptoms and functional status, with the knowledge that if he is not significantly improved, you can add metformin 500 mg twice daily and titrate to 1,000 mg twice daily (see Table 10–5) to assist with avoiding further weight gain and potentially prolong his evolution to full diabetes.

Clinical Pearls: Diabetes

- Though not as sensitive, nonfasting HbA1c can be diagnostic of diabetes and should be obtained whenever blood glucose measurements are taken to screen for diabetes.
- Metformin is always first-line therapy in type 2 diabetes, provided it is tolerated (gastrointestinal side effects usually abate after 1 week) and the patient has no evidence of renal dysfunction (creatinine < 1.5 mg/dL).
- Current HbA1c goals are between 7% and 8%. For individuals who do not achieve this with metformin and a sulfonylurea (glipizide/glyburide), insulin is indicated. A long-acting insulin administered once daily is the first-line choice of insulin therapy.

DYSLIPIDEMIAS

Case Presentation

At the end of his last clinic appointment, you took B.H.'s BP and noted it was elevated at 155/94 mm Hg. Glancing again at his nonfasting labs, you notice his cholesterol values:

- Total cholesterol 220 mg/dL
- High-density lipoprotein (HDL) 34 mg/dL
- Triglycerides 258 mg/dL
- Low-density lipoprotein (LDL) *calculated* 134 mg/dL

These sound high, but you can't remember what the cutoffs are for cholesterol, and you know this was not fasting. You wonder:

- Does B.H. have high cholesterol, and does it put him at risk for CVD?
- Can I use these labs to diagnose high cholesterol or monitor treatment?
- What can I do to help B.H. address his cholesterol values?

Background and Significance

Persons with schizophrenia and bipolar illness are more likely to have abnormal cholesterol profiles (De Hert et al. 2011). In particular, women with schizophrenia are much more likely to have elevated triglycerides and non-HDL cholesterol, which may place them in a separate category of risk (McEvoy et al. 2005). Data from the Clinical Antipsychotic Trials of Intervention Effectiveness (CATIE) indicate that while dyslipidemias are very prevalent among those with SMI, more than 80% go untreated (Nasrallah et al. 2006).

Cholesterol can enter the body through direct ingestion or synthesis from dietary fats, especially saturated and trans fats. A significant proportion of cholesterol found in the body is synthesized in the liver during fasting states (overnight). The rate-limiting step of cholesterol synthesis is the enzyme HMG-CoA reductase, which is inhibited by the popular statin drugs. Cholesterol is transported to tissues through the bloodstream via water-soluble proteins named for their density. High concentrations of LDL have been causally linked to heart attacks and strokes and are an integral component to atherosclerotic plaque formation (Di Angelantonio et al. 2009; Expert Panel on Detection, Evaluation, and Treatment of High Blood Cholesterol in Adults 2001; Stone et al. 2013). These plaques accumulate in arteries and eventually rupture, leading to acute myocardial infarction or ischemic stroke. Reduction in LDL cholesterol has been shown to reduce risk of death and nonfatal myocardial infarction (Expert Panel on Detection, Evaluation, and Treatment of High Blood Cholesterol in Adults 2001; Stone et al. 2013), and cholesterol is one of the leading modifiable risk factors for heart attack and stroke among Americans.

Screening and Diagnosis of Dyslipidemias

Current recommendations from the U.S. Preventive Services Task Force suggest screening adults for dyslipidemia with a fasting lipid panel beginning at age 35 for men and 45 for women (U.S. Preventive Services Task Force 2008). Adults who are obese, have high BP, use tobacco, or have diabetes are candidates for screening beginning at age 20. The American Diabetes Association/American Psychiatric Association consensus panel recommends baseline, 3-month, and every 5 years lipid profiles for adults starting second-generation antipsychotic therapy (American Diabetes Association et al. 2004) (Table 10–2), although many experts believe that adults with abnormal baseline or 3-month values should have their cholesterol checked yearly while receiving antipsychotic treatment, and Table 10–2 has been modified to reflect this change in consensus. Additionally, adults experiencing a gain of over 7% of body weight within 3 months while undergoing therapy should have their cholesterol checked. Given these guidelines, it is estimated that more than 60% of adults seeking care in community mental health centers would qualify for cholesterol screening (Correll et al. 2010).

An individual is diagnosed with high cholesterol when the risk of an intervention (usually with a statin medication) is outweighed by the benefit in reducing their chances of a stroke or myocardial infarction through cholesterol lowering. For individuals with existing CVD, peripheral artery disease, or cerebrovascular disease, the benefit of statin medications generally outweighs the risk and should be started regardless of serum LDL levels up until the age of 75 (Table 10–6, row 1). Persons with diabetes between the ages of 40 and 75 with serum LDL concentrations greater than 70 mg/dL should also be diagnosed with a dyslipidemia and treated accordingly (Table 10–6, row 3).

Non-HDL cholesterol (*total cholesterol minus HDL cholesterol*) levels greater than 220 mg/dL or LDL levels greater than 190 mg/dL are recognized as high enough to warrant intervention regardless of risk or age (Table 10–6, row 2), and a workup of potential secondary causes of dyslipidemias should be undertaken (Table 10–7) (Stone et al. 2013).

For individuals without markedly elevated cholesterol or prior history of CVD, 10-year risk for a major CVD event should be assessed. To appropriately assess risk, total cholesterol and HDL cholesterol must be known, as well as the person's age, smoking status, the presence or absence of diabetes, whether he or she is on therapy for hypertension, and his or her most recent systolic BP. LDL cholesterol is often the focus of clinical attention but requires a fasting laboratory draw if it is calculated *indirectly* (as in our case example). Alternatively, nonfasting non-HDL cholesterol measurement is similarly valid and less costly and should be the preferred measure of unhealthy cholesterol for adults in safety net settings who may have difficulty returning fasting. Estimation of 10-year risk and identification of significantly high cholesterol warranting intervention can be accomplished by obtaining the HDL cholesterol and total cholesterol values, neither of which vary much by fasting status (Sidhu and Naugler 2012). Screening for lipid disorders in adult populations with poor potential for follow-up should therefore include nonfasting triglycerides, HDL, total cholesterol, and alanine transaminase and an HbA1c to determine diabetes status. Calculated LDL cholesterol values may be inappropriately low if nonfasting, are expensive to measure directly, and are not necessary to ascertain risk or prescribe treatment. According to the most recent guidelines, individuals over 40 years of age with a 10-year risk of CVD greater than 7.5%, based in part on their total and HDL cholesterol values, would also benefit from statin therapy (Table 10–6, row 4). Newer calculators for estimating 10-year risk can be accessed online at http://my.americanheart.org/professional/StatementsGuidelines/PreventionGuidelines/Prevention-Guidelines_UCM_457698_SubHomePage.jsp.

Updated guidelines have removed prior LDL targets. Multiple randomized controlled trials have indicated that the intensity of statin therapy is the primary predictor of reduction in stroke or myocardial infarction (Stone et al. 2013) (Table 10–6). Alternative cholesterol-lowering therapies such as fibrates, niacin, ezetimibe, or omega-3 acids have not conclusively demonstrated reductions in morbidity and mortality when lowering blood cholesterol and are not currently standard of care.

Although elevated triglycerides are a risk factor for CVD, targeted triglyceride-lowering therapy has not been conclusively shown to reduce risk of heart attack or stroke. Fasting triglyceride levels above 500 mg/dL warrant focused therapy to reduce the risk of pancreatitis. Interventions for intermediate fasting triglyceride levels (greater than 150 mg/dL and less than 500 mg/dL) should focus on weight loss and treatment with a statin if indicated.

Treatment of Dyslipidemias

Diet and Lifestyle Modification

Treatment of dyslipidemias is typically initiated through intensive diet and lifestyle therapies with reassessment at 3 months. Individuals should strive to achieve diets with less than 7% saturated fat content, 0 g of trans fat, less than 200 mg of exogenous cholesterol intake, and more than 25 g/day of dietary fiber to significantly lower their cholesterol (Kelly 2010; Van Horn et al. 2008). Exercise has also been shown to lower cholesterol, as well as specialized diets rich in Chinese red yeast rice extract and Mediterranean-style foods (Liu et al. 2006). It should be noted that cholesterol lowering by lifestyle intervention, even when intense, usually fails to result in reductions of total or LDL cholesterol greater than 30%, which would be associated with low- to moderate-intensity statin therapy.

TABLE 10–6. Four clinical classes of statin eligibility

Clinical characteristic	Type of prevention	Applicable age range (years)	Preferred statin intensity	Additional Actions
Clinical presence of ASCVD[a]	Secondary	21–75	High	—
Serum LDL >190 mg/dL	Primary	21–75	High	Work up potential secondary causes[b]
Type 2 diabetes[c]	Primary	40–75	Moderate to high	—
10-year risk >7.5%[c]	Primary	40–75	Moderate	—

Note. Dash indicates no additional action to be taken.
[a]Atherosclerotic cardiovascular disease (ASCVD) includes prior myocardial infarction, peripheral vascular disease, stable or unstable angina, abdominal aortic aneurysm, and cerebrovascular disease (ischemic stroke).
[b]Primary prevention takes place when there is no clinical evidence of disease. Secondary prevention applies to therapies in place after the clinical presence of disease.
[c]These recommendations apply to individuals with low-density lipoprotein (LDL) cholesterol values >70 mg/dl..
Source. Adapted from Stone et al. 2013.

TABLE 10–7.   Leading secondary causes of severely elevated blood cholesterol

Secondary cause	Details
Disease/medical/genetic	Type 2 diabetes
	Hypothyroidism
	Chronic kidney disease
	Nephropathy, proteinuria
	Familial (genetic) hyperlipidemia
	Pregnancy[a]
Substance use	Excessive alcohol intake
Medications	Estrogen
	HIV antiretroviral therapy
	Antipsychotic medications
	Steroids, immunosuppressants
Diet	Extreme obesity
	High saturated and trans fats

Note.   [a]Pregnancy and lactation are contraindications to statin therapies.
Source.   Stone et al. 2013; Vodnala et al. 2012.

Pharmacotherapy

Because controlled trials have shown benefit only for statin therapies, they have become the primary means of pharmacological cholesterol risk reduction for the majority of the population. Persons with moderate to severe congestive heart failure and persons on hemodialysis for renal failure have not been shown to benefit from statin therapy and are an exception to this rule. Statin therapies can be divided into high-, moderate-, or low-intensity based on their potency, dose, and potential for lowering LDL (Table 10–8). Greater than 50% reduction in LDL is considered high-intensity therapy, while less than 30% reduction is low-intensity.

Statins are safe and effective in lowering CVD risk among both the general population and the population with SMI (De Hert et al. 2006). Many statins with shorter half-lives are most effective when taken in the evening to prevent fasting synthesis of cholesterol overnight (atorvastatin and rosuvastatin have longer half-lives and may be administered at any time throughout the day). Statins can be safely used in persons with comorbid liver disease, such as hepatitis C, nonalcoholic steatohepatitis, or cirrhosis, as long as baseline transaminase elevations are not greater than 3 times their upper limit of normal (Andrus and East 2010; Gillett and Norrell 2011). For this reason, baseline transaminase assessment is recommended prior to initiation of therapy. In individuals with no known liver disease, regular monitoring of liver function beyond baseline is not necessary. Individuals exhibiting painful myalgias while on a statin should hold off on their treatment, and serum creatinine-kinase

TABLE 10–8. Statin intensity classification by dose and type

Intensity class	LDL cholesterol effect	Drug/daily dosage	Notes
High	≥50% reduction	Atorvastatin 40–80 mg[a] Rosuvastatin 20–40 mg[b]	Higher potency is associated with higher rates of myalgias, side effects
Moderate	30%–50% reduction	Atorvastatin 10 mg[a] Rosuvastatin 5–10 mg[b] Simvastatin 20–40 mg[a] Pravastatin 40–80 mg[b] Lovastatin 40 mg[a] Fluvastatin 40 mg twice daily Pitavastatin 2–4 mg[b]	
Low	<30% reduction	Simvastatin 10 mg[a] Pravastatin 10–20 mg[b] Lovastatin 20 mg[a] Fluvastatin 20–40 mg Pitavastatin 1 mg[b]	Should be reserved for those intolerant of high- to moderate-intensity therapies

Note. LDL=low-density lipoprotein.
[a]Metabolized by CYP3A4, grapefruit juice could raise drug levels, potential interactions with selected other therapies.
[b]No cytochrome P450 metabolism, potentially fewer drug-drug interactions.
Source. Cupp 2012; Stone et al. 2013.

levels should be assessed and the statin discontinued for individuals with levels greater than 3 times the upper limit of normal. Resumption of therapy should be considered on an individual basis, and converting to a lower-dosage or lower-potency statin could be considered.

Treat to Target

Individuals in the highest categories of risk (Table 10–6, rows 1 and 2) should be placed on high-intensity statin therapy as tolerated, and individuals with diabetes or a 10-year risk of CVD greater than 7.5% should be placed on at least a moderate-intensity statin. Individuals with diabetes and a 10-year risk of CVD greater than 7.5% also warrant high-intensity statin therapy. Yearly assessments of total and HDL or LDL cholesterol can aid in reassessing an individual's risk category and ensuring appropriate intensity of statin therapy. Individuals who do not achieve approximate total or LDL cholesterol reduction (≥50% for high intensity, 30%–50% for moderate intensity) after 3 months of therapy should be assessed for adherence or secondary causes of dyslipidemias (Table 10–7). For individuals with no identifiable secondary causes and good adherence, statin therapy should be intensified, and diet and lifestyle interventions should be maximized.

Case Discussion

B.H.'s cholesterol is significantly elevated; his non-HDL cholesterol (total cholesterol minus HDL cholesterol) is 186 mg/dL. Your primary tasks are to engage B.H. in intensive diet and lifestyle modifications and to identify if B.H. is a candidate for statin therapy, which intensity level to assign him to (high or moderate), and when to begin therapy. B.H. is 46 years old and has no history of CVD or strokes. B.H.'s calculated LDL value given in the beginning of the chapter is nonfasting and likely underestimates his true LDL value. However, assuming it is unlikely his actual LDL cholesterol is extremely high, or above 190 mg/dL (which would warrant high-intensity statin therapy automatically), and given that his non-HDL cholesterol is less than 220 mg/dL (a viable nonfasting substitute), you navigate to an online risk calculator (http://my.americanheart.org/professional/StatementsGuidelines/PreventionGuidelines/Prevention-Guidelines_UCM_457698_SubHomePage.jsp) and put in his risk factors. He comes out at a 14.4% risk of having a heart attack or stroke in the next 10 years, which is above the cutoff of 7.5%. He doesn't have diabetes. B.H. has already started to try walking and switching to diet soda, and you recently made the switch to aripiprazole, so you decide to not make any adjustments and see if these initial interventions are helpful.

After 3 months of this, he comes back to clinic and repeats some nonfasting labs, which show an HbA1c of 6.1% and a non-HDL cholesterol of 205 mg/dL. Because his 10-year risk is still above 7.5%, you and B.H. decide to start atorvastatin 20 mg, a moderate-intensity therapy (Table 10–8), acknowledging there is a potential interaction with his risperidone injection because of cytochrome P450 inhibition. You choose atorvastatin because he can take it once a day in the morning with his aripiprazole, and he needs a greater than 30% reduction in cholesterol (at least moderate therapy), which may not be possible with a less potent statin such as pravastatin. You will monitor his risperidone and perhaps adjust down the dose of his injection over time if he tolerates the switch to aripiprazole well (he has so far).

Clinical Pearls: Dyslipidemias

- Many statins are metabolized through the liver cytochrome P450 system and may increase levels of psychotherapeutics. Pravastatin is generic and may not have the drug-drug interactions inherent with other statins but may be less effective in lowering LDL cholesterol substantially.
- Recent cholesterol guidelines emphasize the goal of therapy is tolerance of a statin medication at the most appropriate level of intensity instead of traditional cholesterol targets.

- Rosuvastatin and atorvastatin are among the most potent statins and are available once daily for individuals with poor adherence patterns.

HYPERTENSION

Case Presentation

You noted at B.H.'s last appointment that in addition to his glucose intolerance, morbid obesity, and high cholesterol, he also has hypertension. When you measured his BP in your office at the last visit, 3 months prior, it was 155/94 mm Hg. At this follow-up visit, he's had 3 months to try and start walking and switching to diet soda, and he's symptom-stable on aripiprazole 20 mg/day. He's lost about 4 lbs, and you note that his BP is still elevated at 156/95 mm Hg. You recall that his labs from 3 months ago demonstrated normal serum electrolytes, including creatinine of 0.91 mg/dL. You wonder:

- When does he need a medication to treat his BP?
- What type of medication should be used to treat his hypertension?

Background and Significance

Multiple longitudinal studies have linked hypertension to stroke and myocardial infarction and subsequent lowering of hypertension to reductions in morbidity and mortality (Chobanian et al. 2003). In adults with SMI, rates of hypertension range between 20% and 60% (De Hert et al. 2011). Such high prevalence is likely due to higher rates of obesity, smoking, alcohol and substance use, sedentary lifestyle, and use of some medications (including serotonin-norepinephrine reuptake inhibitors, stimulants, and second-generation antipsychotics). Despite the relative ease of measurement and highly effective therapies, treatment of hypertension among adults with SMI remains stubbornly low and warrants more aggressive attention (Nasrallah et al. 2006).

Screening and Diagnosis of High Blood Pressure

All adults are eligible for BP screening beginning at age 18 and for those with no risk factors (e.g., obesity, smoking, atypical antipsychotic use) and values less than 120 mm Hg systolic or 80 mm Hg diastolic every 2 years thereafter. Table 10–2 indicates the regular screening protocols for BP in adults on atypical antipsychotics, and BP should be monitored at least yearly for adults who are overweight (BMI 25 or greater) or smoke (U.S. Preventive Services Task Force 2003). For adults on a stable BP regimen or with known hypertension, monitoring every 3–6 months, or even yearly, may be acceptable once they reach adequate control.

BP measurement should be taken with the patient sitting upright, with an appropriately sized cuff over the brachial artery at the level of the heart after the patient has been resting for several minutes, preferably at least 60 minutes since the use of tobacco products or caffeine. High readings should be repeated after at least 5 minutes (perhaps at the end of the appointment) and confirmed. Alternatives to office-based measurements are becoming increasingly common and trade convenience for reliability and validity. Persons should be encouraged to obtain home- or pharmacy-based BP measurements using an appropriate device, and discrepancies in results can be addressed by calibrating their device against one maintained in a clinical setting. BPs obtained each morning after awakening and each evening before going to bed for 3 consecutive days are fairly accurate and can approximate a continuous 24-hour ambulatory BP monitor (Hodgkinson et al. 2011).

Hypertension cutoffs are listed in Table 10–9 according to specific disease states or demographics. Generally, if either systolic BP exceeds 140 mm Hg or diastolic BP exceeds 90 mm Hg after repeated measurements over 1 week apart, the person may be diagnosed with hypertension. Adults more than 60 years of age should have a target BP of 150 mm Hg systolic and 90 mm Hg diastolic (James et al. 2014). Only 5%–10% of ambulatory hypertension is secondary to an identifiable cause (secondary hypertension), of which renovascular disease, obstructive sleep apnea, and primary aldosteronism are the most common (Viera and Neutze 2010). Because the vast majority of hypertension is essential, or primary, most persons with elevated BP can be tried on up to three pharmacotherapies before secondary workup is warranted (Calhoun et al. 2008). Individuals whose BP is not controlled after three medications warrant close evaluation of adherence and potentially a secondary workup. Persons under the age of 18 require initial workup for secondary causes (Viera and Neutze 2010).

Stage 2 hypertension is systolic BP above 160 mm Hg or diastolic BP above 100 mm Hg. Control of stage 2 hypertension typically requires two or more (combination) pharmacotherapies but can be managed safely in ambulatory settings (Chobanian et al. 2003). Hypertensive emergencies are rare but are defined as the presence of end-organ damage usually in the context of severe hypertension. End-organ damage is the presence of ischemic changes on a 12-lead electrocardiogram, headache or focal neurologic symptoms, changes or loss of vision, or laboratory evidence of renal insufficiency (elevated serum creatinine) and requires emergent evaluation and treatment.

Treatment of Hypertension

Diet and Lifestyle Modification

Nonpharmacologic management of hypertension should be part of treatment. Low-salt diets, moderation of alcohol use, weight loss, and smoking cessation have all been shown to lower BP, and effects are almost equivalent

TABLE 10–9. Target blood pressure and preferred medications by clinical presentation

Patient	Goal SBP/DBP (mm Hg)	Medical notes and preferred agents
Normal	<140/<90	Thiazide diuretic or CCB (amlodipine) first-line
Adults ≥ 60 years	<150/<90	Adults tolerating lower BPs may maintain successful regimens, but polypharmacy should be minimized.
Diabetes	140/90	ACE inhibitor/ARB if CKD present, otherwise CCB or diuretic may be first-line
Congestive heart failure/post–myocardial infarction	130/90	Beta-blocker first-line, including carvedilol (alpha and beta)
End-stage renal disease	140/90	ACE inhibitor/ARB if tolerated Cr
African American	140/90	Consider amlodipine and diuretic first-line

Note. ACE=angiotensin converting enzyme; ARB=angiotensin II receptor blocker; BP=blood pressure; CCB=calcium channel blocker; CKD=chronic kidney disease; Cr=creatinine; DBP=diastolic blood pressure; SBP=systolic blood pressure.
ACE inhibitors and ARBs should be held if hyperkalemia cannot be controlled or for a persistent rise above baseline serum creatinine >30%.
Source. Adapted from James et al. 2014.

(5–10 mm Hg) to those of pharmacologic therapies, but they may be harder to maintain (Appel et al. 2006). The following link provides instructions for the popular DASH diet, which has been demonstrated to significantly lower BP: http://dashdiet.org/.

Pharmacotherapy

Pharmacotherapy for hypertension is safe and effective when monitored appropriately. First-line agents include thiazide diuretics (e.g., hydrochlorothiazide or chlorthalidone), ACE inhibitors (e.g., lisinopril), and ARBs (e.g., losartan) or dihydropyridine calcium channel blockers (e.g., amlodipine) (James et al. 2013). Diuretics should not be used in individuals at risk of significant drug-drug interactions (e.g., those on lithium therapy). In the absence of a clear indication for a particular class of medication (such as ACE inhibitors for patients with diabetes or chronic kidney disease or beta-blockers for those with congestive heart failure; Table 10–9) (Jamerson and Weber 2008; James et al. 2014), calcium channel blockers such as amlodipine may be the preferred first-line agent in the population with SMI because of their ease of use, efficacy, relative lack of drug-drug interactions, and lack of need for follow-up electrolyte or renal function testing. Additionally, if it is suspected that combination therapy will be required to control BP (as is frequently the case), an ACE or ARB and amlodipine is the preferred combination (Jamerson and Weber 2008).

Many antihypertensive combination pills are available in generic formulations now, easing both the cost of treatment and adherence to multidrug regimens. Table 10–10 lists common BP medications, their dosage ranges, monitoring guidelines, drug-drug interactions, and frequent side effects (combination therapies are highly variable by region and formulary and are not listed). Lithium levels should be monitored closely (at least at initiation and every 3 months until stable) in individuals taking ACE inhibitors or ARBs and diuretics.

Treat to Target

The magnitude of BP reduction is more important than the type of pharmacological agent chosen for reducing CVD risk. For this reason, when therapy is initiated, treatment tracking and follow-up are critical to ensuring therapeutic goals (Table 10–9). If hypertensive goals are not sustained after documented adherence to three maximum-dose therapies (usually an ACE/ARB, thiazide diuretic, and calcium channel blocker), an evaluation for secondary causes of hypertension should be undertaken. ACE and ARB therapies should not be used simultaneously because they have a similar mechanism of action. Alternative classes of BP-lowering medications, such as beta-blockers, aldosterone antagonists (spironolactone), or clonidine, could then be entertained (James et al. 2014). This usually requires referral to primary care or a hypertension specialist.

Case Discussion

B.H.'s BP has never been above 160 mm Hg systolic, though it's close. B.H.'s target BP, given no history of congestive heart failure, is less than 140 mm Hg systolic and less than 90 mm Hg diastolic. You decide for simplicity to start a single agent, and you choose chlorthalidone 12.5 mg once daily. (If he had diabetes, you would have chosen an ACE inhibitor such as benazepril, and if his BP were greater than 160 mm Hg, you might have started him on a combination of amlodipine and an ACE inhibitor or ARB.) B.H. comes back in 2 weeks, and while his BP is lower (144/88), it is still not at goal (less than 140 mm Hg systolic), and his potassium is now 3.3 mg/dL, down from 4.5 mg/dL before starting chlorthalidone. To help spare his potassium and further reduce his BP, you add benazepril 10 mg/day because it can help preserve potassium. In retrospect, you might have started him on just amlodipine to avoid a potential complication with hypokalemia, and you remember that for next time.

He now takes atorvastatin 20 mg, benazepril 10 mg, chlorthalidone 12.5 mg, and aripiprazole 20 mg every morning in addition to his risperidone injection.

TABLE 10–10. Details on selected blood pressure medications

Class	Medication, dosage	Laboratory monitoring	Drug interactions	Side effects	Contraindications
Thiazide diuretics	Hydrochlorothiazide, 12.5–50 mg once daily Chlorthalidone (preferred), 12.5–25 mg once daily	Potassium levels 1 week after initiation of therapy	Increases serum lithium levels	Increased urination Stomach upset	Hypokalemia Gout Osteoporosis
ACE inhibitors	Benazepril (preferred), 10–40 mg once daily Lisinopril, 10–40 mg once daily	Potassium and Cr levels 1 week after initiation of therapy, periodically thereafter	May increase serum lithium levels	Dry cough Angioedema Elevated potassium levels	Pregnancy Preexisting kidney disease
Angiotensin II receptor blockers	Losartan, 25–100 mg once or twice daily Irbesartan, 150–300 mg once daily Valsartan, 80–320 mg once or twice daily	Potassium and Cr levels 1 week after initiation of therapy, periodically thereafter	May increase serum lithium levels	Elevated potassium levels	Pregnancy Preexisting kidney disease
Calcium channel blockers—dihydropyridines	Amlodipine 2.5–10 mg once daily	None necessary	Little effect on lithium	Headache Lower extremity swelling	

TABLE 10–10. Details on selected blood pressure medications *(continued)*

Class	Medication, dosage	Laboratory monitoring	Drug interactions	Side effects	Contraindications
Beta-blockers (third-line agents)	Atenolol (preferred), 25–100 mg once daily Metoprolol (XL), 50–100 mg once or twice daily (once for XL) Propranolol, 40–160 mg twice daily Carvedilol (combination alpha and beta), 3.125–25 mg twice daily	Pulse	Watch for CYP2D6 interactions	Fatigue Cold hands Headache Constipation Depression	Severe reactive airway disease (asthma)

Note. Cr= creatinine; CYP2D6=cytochrome P450 2D6.

His pharmacy has helped by providing him with a pillbox. He returns in another 2 weeks, and his potassium and creatinine are normal, he is having no side effects, and his BP is now 135/85.

Clinical Pearls: Hypertension

- While diuretics have traditionally been first-line therapy, consideration should be given to amlodipine for ease of use and reduction of possible drug-drug interactions in the population with SMI.
- Individuals with BP exceeding 160 mm Hg systolic should be initially offered combination therapy with two BP agents to improve their chances of attaining successful lowering.
- If an individual is adherent to three BP therapies at appropriate doses and has not reached goal, he or she needs referral and workup for refractory hypertension.

TOBACCO USE DISORDERS

Case Presentation

After 4 months of working with B.H., you have his BP under better control and his elevated cholesterol and glucose values are being worked on, but today you see the nicotine stains on his fingers and beard and are reminded of the heavy amount of tobacco he uses. When you ask him about it, he says that he rolls his own cigarettes, smoking one about every 20–30 minutes when he's awake (times 14 hours, this is about 28/day). He does this because he feels it's healthier (more natural), and it's also cheaper to buy the tobacco in bulk. Since he's 46 years old, and he says he's been smoking since he was 16 years old, you estimate around 60 pack-years of tobacco use. He has tried to quit on several occasions, and at one point was successful going "cold turkey" for 6 months when he was in a state hospital, but he has not tried for years. B.H. says that if he didn't smoke, he is not sure what he would do to pass the time and notes that now is a particularly stressful time in his life. You wonder:

- Can B.H. successfully stop smoking?
- Will smoking cessation impact his mental illness or have an effect on his medications?
- Are cessation medications safe or even effective for B.H.?

Background and Significance

Tobacco use–related disorders are responsible for as much as half of the premature mortality and morbidity of those with severe and persistent mental illness and by some estimates are the leading cause of cardiovascular mortality in the United States (Callaghan et al. 2014; Critchley and Capewell

2003). As tobacco cessation efforts in recent decades have curbed prevalence rates among the general population, those with SMI maintain high rates of tobacco use, resulting in widening health disparities (Dickerson et al. 2013). For further background on tobacco use in the population with SMI, refer to Chapter 7.

Screening and Diagnosis of Tobacco Use Disorders

All adults in the general population should be asked at regular intervals about exposure to nicotine (i.e., every office visit) (Calonge et al. 2009). There is less evidence for population-based screening of youth; however, those enrolled in mental health care should be evaluated for concurrent substance use, including nicotine, as part of their routine examination. The type and amount of daily nicotine consumption should be ascertained, as well as prior quit attempts and methods and current transtheoretical stage of change (precontemplative, contemplative, action, or maintenance) (DiClemente et al. 1991).

There are a number of evidence-based methods to inquire about tobacco use in clinical settings, including mental health settings. These interventions are usually based on the screening, brief intervention, and referral to treatment (SBIRT) model of care, similar to the five As approach recommended by the U.S. Preventive Services Task Force. The five As refer to five steps of tobacco intervention: 1) ask permission to inquire about tobacco use, 2) assess amount of use, 3) advise the patient on the harmful effects of tobacco use, 4) offer assistance in quitting, and 5) arrange a referral or clinical follow-up. Additionally, the implementation of a system for tracking tobacco users, clinician education and feedback to improve evidence-based interventions, and the provision of dedicated staff (such as peers, nurses, case managers) to oversee tobacco-related programming are all effective methods for curtailing tobacco use (Fiore 2008).

Those with any tobacco usage are at increased risk of medical morbidity and mortality at any age. Screening instruments employing exhaled carbon monoxide levels can help identify and track nicotine use, providing point-of-care teaching resources for persons ambivalent about engaging in smoking cessation. Systematic reviews of biomedical risk assessment (carbon monoxide monitors) show weak evidence for these types of interventions above the usual strategies listed above in the population with SMI and likely offer little advantage over patient self-report (Bize et al. 2012; Rose and Behm 2013).

Treatment of Tobacco Use Disorders

Pharmacotherapy: Nicotine Replacement

The cornerstone of tobacco cessation is nicotine replacement therapy (NRT). Though ideally it should be coupled with counseling, the effect sizes seen across the forms of nicotine replacement are similar regardless of the form or presence of counseling (Stead et al. 2012). The average dose of nicotine is approximately 1 mg per cigarette smoked, with a one-pack-per-day habit being approximately equal to a daily dose of 20 mg of nicotine. Forms of nicotine replacement can and should be combined and tailored to approximate at least 80% of the current daily usage of patients attempting to quit to foster the greatest chance of success. A person smoking in excess of one pack per day should be considered for combination therapy with a 21-mg patch and a second patch or gum or lozenges or inhalers timed to address breakthrough cravings (Williams and Foulds 2007). Combination forms of NRT have been proven safe and effective beyond monotherapies, especially in adults with multiple failed quit attempts, which may be common in the psychiatric population. Starting NRT 2 weeks leading up to a quit date may also improve chances at a successful quit attempt (Rose and Behm 2013). NRT can also be safely used through smoking relapse or with concurrent smoking and significantly improves chances of cessation when used more consistently (Zapawa et al. 2011). Individuals starting at the 21-mg patch/day level may continue on that for the first 6 weeks of therapy, then step down to the 14-mg level for 2 weeks, followed by the 7-mg level for 2 weeks, for a total of 10 weeks of therapy. Though this is the current recommendation, some experts believe continued use of NRT beyond formal guidelines if abstinence is obtained is less harmful than gradual taper and potential relapse. It should be noted that the monthly cost of NRT is about equivalent to the cost of smoking 1 pack per day over a month (Table 10–11).

Pharmacotherapy: Non-Nicotine Replacement

Either augmentation or monotherapy with the U.S. Food and Drug Administration–approved pharmaceuticals bupropion XL or varenicline has been proven safe and effective in patients with schizophrenia, though more limited data exist for those with mood spectrum illnesses (Cerimele and Durango 2012; Rose and Behm 2013; Williams and Anthenelli 2012). In one trial, patients with schizophrenia who were randomly assigned to varenicline had no difference in psychotic symptoms or adverse events compared to control subjects (Williams and Anthenelli 2012). A recent large review found little evidence in support of NRT for those with schizophrenia, but only one trial in the review examined the role of combination NRT, which may be necessary to address the higher rates of nicotine consumption in those with psychotic illnesses (Tsoi et al. 2013). Table 10–11 lists the common pharmacological agents used in smoking cessation and their dosage guidelines, approximate cost, side effects, and monitoring parameters. At the very least, persons with SMI who smoke should be offered pharmacotherapy and counseling depending on their preference and the absence of contraindications.

TABLE 10–11. Pharmacotherapy for tobacco cessation

Class	Medication, dosage	Cost per day/ week/month[a]	Laboratory monitoring	Drug interactions	Side effects	Practical pointers	Contraindications
NRT	Nicotine patch 7–21 mg/day transdermal Start 21 mg/day for 6 weeks, then 14 mg for 2 weeks, then 7 mg for 2 weeks	$20–$50/week, $80–$200/ month	None	None	Skin irritation Nightmares in some patients when worn overnight	Put on after showering. Remove daily. Sweaty persons should be prepared with extra adhesive supplies; hairy people may require shaving.	Intolerance of topical preparation, excessive sweating
NRT	Nicotine lozenge 2–4 mg every 1–2 hours as needed for craving Nicotine gum 2–4 mg every 1–2 hours as needed for craving	Lozenge: $6–$12/day, $180–$360/ month Gum: $240/ month	None	None	Local mucosal inflammation	Gum is chewed and then allowed to rest in cheek to aid absorption.	None

TABLE 10–11. Pharmacotherapy for tobacco cessation (*continued*)

Class	Medication, dosage	Cost per day/ week/month[a]	Laboratory monitoring	Drug interactions	Side effects	Practical pointers	Contraindications
NRT	Nicotine inhaler 20–40 puffs over 20 minutes, to be repeated as needed for cravings throughout the day Nicotine nasal spray 1–5 puffs over 1 hour as needed for cravings	Available as a prescription, copays vary dramatically by plan. Talk to pharmacist.	None	None	Oral mucosal irritation Headache Possible nicotine toxicity	Inhaler puff should be held in the mouth (not inhaled) for absorption. Inhaler may not extinguish behavioral cues (hand-mouth reinforcement). Nasal spray may deliver more concentrated doses than necessary in the population with SMI.	Those with severe breathing problems, hypersensitivity to device/drug

TABLE 10–11. Pharmacotherapy for tobacco cessation *(continued)*

Class	Medication, dosage	Cost per day/ week/month[a]	Laboratory monitoring	Drug interactions	Side effects	Practical pointers	Contraindications
Pharmaceutical, non-NRT	Bupropion SR/XL Start 150 mg/day 2 weeks prior to quit date, then increase as tolerated to 300 mg/day	Available as a prescription, copays vary dramatically by plan. Talk to pharmacist.	No lab monitoring necessary, monitor mood/ anxiety/ sleep and irritability	Few to none	Jitters Anxiety Sleeplessness	Optimal doses are ~300 mg/day.	Eating disorders, seizure disorders
Pharmaceutical, non-NRT	Varenicline Begin 1 week prior to quit date, days 1–3: 0.5 mg daily, then days 4–7: 0.5 mg twice daily, then days >8: 1 mg twice daily (Many pharmacies accept prescriptions for "varenicline starter packs" as a substitute for the exact initiation regimen.)	Available as a prescription, copays vary dramatically by plan. Talk to pharmacist.	Mood, suicidal ideation	Few to none (nicotine partial agonist)	Nausea Insomnia Headache	Second-line choice for population with SMI. Do not combine with NRT.	Mood spectrum illness, actively suicidal

Note. NRT = nicotine replacement therapy; SMI = serious mental illness.
[a]Compare with average cost of smoking 1 pack/day in 2013: $6.74/day, $47/week, $189/month (www.theawl.com/2011/06/what-a-pack-of-cigarettes-costs-state-by-state).

The tar (not nicotine) in cigarette smoke has been associated with cytochrome P450 enzyme induction and consequently lowers levels of some common antipsychotics, primarily haloperidol, olanzapine, and clozapine. Dose reductions of those psychotropics in particular may be necessary if abstinence or significant reductions in cigarette smoking are attained (Desai et al. 2001; Williams and Foulds 2007). Some antipsychotics such as clozapine have been associated with significant reductions in tobacco consumption because of agonist potential at the nicotinic acid receptor (Freedman et al. 2000). This may explain some variance in the therapeutic benefit of clozapine for refractory schizophrenia (Williams and Foulds 2007).

Treat to Target

Longitudinal tracking measures for use in tobacco cessation have not been systematically reviewed. In general, risk decreases as early as 1 year postcessation, but even minimal amounts of tobacco consumption are associated with large increases in mortality from lung cancer or heart disease (Critchley and Capewell 2003). Though any reduction in tobacco use is laudable, persistent efforts should be made to see cessation attempts through to complete abstinence.

Case Discussion

After you ask B.H. about his smoking habits, he states that he knows it is not healthy for him to smoke, that it still costs a lot every week (even to roll his own), and that he has an annoying cough on occasion. After further discussion, he decides he is ready to try quitting again and wants some assistance. He has benefited from the nicotine patch in the past. You set a quit date with him for an upcoming major holiday and agree to start bupropion SR 150 mg 2 weeks prior and plan on titrating up to 300 mg, divided twice daily for the SR form or once daily in XL form, in combination with a high-dose nicotine patch (21 mg). You then arrange to have his case manager, who is facile with tobacco cessation counseling, touch base a week after the holiday to see if he's enacted the plan, and you make a note to follow up with his results at your next appointment in a month.

At that appointment, he's reduced his smoking to only when he's having a major craving, which occurs about twice a day (first thing in the morning, dinnertime/evening). He's tolerating bupropion XL 300 mg/day well. You decide to add nicotine gum at the time of his cravings and follow up in another month.

Clinical Pearls: Tobacco Cessation

- Combinations of NRT can improve the chances of clinical cessation, especially in those who have failed cessation before.

- NRT should be continued through relapse and improves chances at full cessation if use is maintained.
- Both bupropion and varenicline have been proven safe and effective in adults with SMI.

CONCLUSION

B.H.'s case highlights many of the health disparities in the population with SMI, primarily cardiovascular risks. By systematically managing all of his risks in this chapter, you have assisted B.H. in lowering his overall 10-year risk of a heart attack or stroke from 15% to 4%, a dramatic reduction. For every 10 patients like B.H. who similarly lower their risk, you are preventing one from death or heart attack in 10 years. B.H.'s overall risk for CVD was only reduced when there was systematic follow-up and achievement of goals in his chronic disease care. Whenever possible, threats to health and well-being should be communicated to patients so they may be empowered to make their own decisions regarding their choices in pursuing healthy lifestyles. In B.H.'s case, when given choices, he frequently chose to pursue a healthier life, though this may not always be the case. Mental health practitioners are uniquely suited to have these conversations with their patients and may be pleasantly surprised to find many interested in seeking wellness through a variety of methods.

The widening mortality gap of persons with SMI is multifactorial but appears to be driven by premature cardiovascular mortality. Clinicians interested in addressing these disparities in care should familiarize themselves with the evidence-based approaches to the various risk factors contributing to this excessive mortality and develop the skill sets within their clinical comfort that can allow them to work effectively with primary care colleagues as an integral member of their client's health care team. The information herein could even allow a psychiatrist to manage the leading chronic diseases placing their clients at risk for premature death. Psychiatrists managing cardiovascular risk are encouraged to seek support and collaboration from primary care colleagues to ensure they deliver up-to-date care and have appropriate backup in case referral is necessary. By instituting care reforms that are based on principles outlined in this chapter, clinicians of the future may finally be able to reduce the mortality gap of those with persistent mental illness.

REFERENCES

Ahmed A, Warton E, Schaefer C: The effect of bariatric surgery on psychiatric course among patients with bipolar disorder. Bipolar Disord 15(7):753–763, 2013

Alberti K, Eckel R, Grundy S: Harmonizing the metabolic syndrome: a joint interim statement of the International Diabetes Federation Task Force on Epidemiology and Prevention; National Heart, Lung and Blood Institute; American Heart Association; World Heart Federation; International Atherosclerosis Society; and International Association for the Study of Obesity. Circulation 120:1640–1645, 2009

Ali M, Echouffo-Tcheugui J, Williamson D: How effective were lifestyle interventions in real-world settings that were modeled on the Diabetes Prevention Program? Health Aff (Millwood) 31(1):67–75, 2012

American Diabetes Association: Diagnosis and classification of diabetes mellitus. Diabetes Care 33 (suppl 1):S62–S69, 2010

American Diabetes Association: Standards of medical care in diabetes—2013. Diabetes Care 36 (suppl 1):S11–S66, 2013

American Diabetes Association, American Psychiatric Association, American Association of Clinical Endocrinologists, et al: Consensus Development Conference on Antipsychotic Drugs and Obesity and Diabetes. Diabetes Care 27(2):596–601, 2004

Andrus MR, East J: Use of statins in patients with chronic hepatitis C. South Med J 103(10):1018–1022, quiz 1023, 2010

Appel LJ, Brands MW, Daniels SR, et al: Dietary approaches to prevent and treat hypertension: a scientific statement from the American Heart Association. Hypertension 47(2):296–308, 2006

Becker T, Hux J: Risk of acute complications of diabetes among people with schizophrenia in Ontario, Canada. Diabetes Care 34:398–402, 2011

Bize R, Burnand B, Mueller Y, et al: Biomedical risk assessment as an aid for smoking cessation. Cochrane Database of Systematic Reviews 2012, Issue 12. Art. No.: CD004705. DOI: 10.1002/14651858.CD004705.pub4.

Bonfioli E, Berti L, Goss C, et al: Health promotion lifestyle interventions for weight management in psychosis: a systematic review and meta-analysis of randomised controlled trials. BMC Psychiatry 12:78, 2012

Calhoun D, Jones D, Textor S, et al: Resistant hypertension: diagnosis, evaluation, and treatment: a scientific statement from the American Heart Association Professional Education Committee of the Council for High Blood Pressure Research. Circulation 117(25):e510–e526, 2008

Callaghan RC, Veldhuizen S, Jeysingh T, et al: Patterns of tobacco-related mortality among individuals diagnosed with schizophrenia, bipolar disorder, or depression. J Psychiatr Res 48(1):102–110, 2014

Calonge N, Petitti D, DeWitt T: Counseling and interventions to prevent tobacco use and tobacco-caused disease in adults and pregnant women: U.S. Preventive Services Task Force reaffirmation recommendation statement. Ann Intern Med 150(8):551–556, 2009

Cerimele JM, Durango A: Does varenicline worsen psychiatric symptoms in patients with schizophrenia or schizoaffective disorder? J Clin Psychiatry 73(8):e1039–e1047, 2012

Chiuve SE, Fung TT, Rexrode KM, et al: Adherence to a low-risk, healthy lifestyle and risk of sudden cardiac death among women. JAMA 306(1):62–69, 2011

Chobanian A, Bakris G, Black H: Seventh report of the Joint National Committee on Prevention, Detection, Evaluation, and Treatment of High Blood Pressure. 289(19):2560–2572, 2003

Colton CW, Manderscheid RW: Congruencies in increased mortality rates, years of potential life lost, and causes of death among public mental health clients in eight states. Prev Chronic Dis 3(2):A42, 2006

Correll C, Frederickson A: Metabolic syndrome and the risk of coronary heart disease in 367 patients treated with second-generation antipsychotic drugs. J Clin Psychiatry 67(4):575–583, 2006

Correll C, Druss BG, Lombardo I, et al: Findings of a U.S. national cardiometabolic screening program among 10,084 psychiatric outpatients. Psychiatr Serv 61(9):892–898, 2010

Critchley J, Capewell S: Mortality risk reduction associated with smoking cessation in patients with coronary heart disease. JAMA 290(1):86–97, 2003

Crump C, Sundquist K, Winkleby M, et al: Comorbidities and mortality in bipolar disorder: a Swedish national cohort study. JAMA Psychiatry 70(9):931–939, 2013a

Crump C, Winkleby M, Sundquist K, et al: Comorbidities and mortality in persons with schizophrenia: a Swedish national cohort study. Am J Psychiatry 170(3):324–333, 2013b

Cupp M: Characteristics of the various statins. Pharmacist's Letter 28(6):280606, 2012

Daumit GL, Dickerson FB, Wang N-Y, et al: A behavioral weight-loss intervention in persons with serious mental illness. N Engl J Med 368(17):1594–1602, 2013

De Hert M, Kalnicka D, van Winkel R, et al: Treatment with rosuvastatin for severe dyslipidemia in patients with schizophrenia and schizoaffective disorder. J Clin Psychiatry 67(12):1889–1896, 2006

De Hert M, Correll CU, Bobes J, et al: Physical illness in patients with severe mental disorders, I: prevalence, impact of medications and disparities in health care. World Psychiatry 10(1):52–77, 2011

Desai H, Seabolt J, Jann M: Smoking in patients receiving psychotropic medications: a pharmacokinetic perspective. CNS Drugs 15(6):469–494, 2001

Diabetes Control and Complications Trial/Epidemiology of Diabetes Interventions and Complications (DCCT/EDIC) Study Research Group: Intensive diabetes treatment and cardiovascular disease in patients with type 1 diabetes. N Engl J Med 353(25):2643–2653, 2005

Di Angelantonio E, Sarwar N, Perry P, et al: Major lipids, apolipoproteins, and risk of vascular disease. JAMA 302(18):1993–2000, 2009

Dickerson F, Stallings C, Origoni A: Cigarette smoking among persons with schizophrenia or bipolar disorder in routine clinical settings, 1999–2011. Psychiatr Serv 64(1):44–50, 2013

DiClemente CC, Prochaska JO, Fairhurst SK, et al: The process of smoking cessation: an analysis of precontemplation, contemplation, and preparation stages of change. J Consult Clin Psychol 59(2):295–304, 1991

Dixon J, Zimmet P, Alberti K, et al: Bariatric surgery: an IDF statement for obese type 2 diabetes. Diabet Med 28(6):628–642, 2011

Druss B, Zhao L, Cummings J: Mental comorbidity and quality of diabetes care under Medicaid: a 50-state analysis. Med Care 50(5):428–433, 2012

Expert Panel on Detection, Evaluation, and Treatment of High Blood Cholesterol in Adults: Executive summary of the Third Report of the National Cholesterol Education Program (NCEP) Expert Panel on Detection, Evaluation, and Treatment of High Blood Cholesterol in Adults (Adult Treatment Panel III). JAMA 285(19):2486–2497, 2001

Fagiolini A, Frank E, Scott J: Metabolic syndrome in bipolar disorder: findings from the Bipolar Disorder Center for Pennsylvanians. Bipolar Disord 7:424–430, 2005

Fiore M: Treating Tobacco Use and Dependence: 2008 Update. Baltimore, MD, U.S. Department of Health and Human Services, Public Health Service, 2008

Freedman R, Adams C, Leonard S: The alpha7-nicotinic acetylcholine receptor and the pathology of hippocampal interneurons in schizophrenia. J Chem Neuroanat 20(3–4):299–306, 2000

Gillett RC, Norrell A: Considerations for safe use of statins: liver enzyme abnormalities and muscle toxicity. Am Fam Physician 83(6):711–716, 2011

Goldberg R, Temprosa M, Haffner S: Effect of progression from impaired glucose tolerance to diabetes on cardiovascular risk factors and its amelioration by lifestyle and metformin intervention. Diabetes Care 32(4):726–732, 2009

Goldstein D: Beneficial health effects of modest weight loss. Int J Obes Relat Metab Disord 16(6):397–415, 1992

Hamoui N, Kingsbury S, Anthone GJ, et al: Surgical treatment of morbid obesity in schizophrenic patients. Obes Surg 14(3):349–352, 2004

Hodgkinson J, Mant J, Martin U: Relative effectiveness of clinic and home blood pressure monitoring compared with ambulatory blood pressure monitoring in diagnosis of hypertension: systematic review. BMJ 342:d3621, 2011

International Expert Committee: International Expert Committee report on the role of the A1c assay in the diagnosis of diabetes. Diabetes Care 32(7):1327–1334, 2009

Jamerson K, Weber M: Benazepril plus amlodipine or hydrochlorothiazide for hypertension in high-risk patients. N Engl J Med 359(23):2417–2428, 2008

James PA, Oparil S, Carter BL, et al: 2014 evidence-based guideline for the management of high blood pressure in adults: report from the panel members appointed to the Eighth Joint National Committee (JNC 8). JAMA 311:507–520, 2014

Jarskog LF, Hamer RM, Catellier DJ, et al: Metformin for weight loss and metabolic control in overweight outpatients with schizophrenia and schizoaffective disorder. Am J Psychiatry 170(9):1032–1040, 2013

Kashyap S, Bhatt D, Wolski K: Metabolic effects of bariatric surgery in patients with moderate obesity and type 2 diabetes: analysis of a randomized control trial comparing surgery with intensive medical treatment. Diabetes Care 36(8):2175–2182, 2013

Kelly RB: Diet and exercise in the management of hyperlipidemia. Am Fam Physician 81(9):1097–1102, 2010

Knowler W, Barrett-Connor E, Fowler S, et al: Reduction in the incidence of type II diabetes with lifestyle intervention or metformin. N Engl J Med 346(6):393–403, 2002

Liu J, Zhang J, Shi Y, et al: Chinese red yeast rice (Monascus purpureus) for primary hyperlipidemia: a meta-analysis of randomized controlled trials. Chin Med 1:4, 2006

Maayan L, Vakhrusheva J, Correll CU: Effectiveness of medications used to attenuate antipsychotic-related weight gain and metabolic abnormalities: a systematic review and meta-analysis. Neuropsychopharmacology 35(7):1520–1530, 2010

Mai Q, Holman C, Sanfilippo F: Mental illness related disparities in diabetes prevalence, quality of care and outcomes: a population-based longitudinal study. BMC Psychiatry 9:118–129, 2011

McEvoy JP, Meyer JM, Goff DC, et al: Prevalence of the metabolic syndrome in patients with schizophrenia: baseline results from the Clinical Antipsychotic Trials of Intervention Effectiveness (CATIE) schizophrenia trial and comparison with national estimates from NHANES III. Schizophr Res 80(1):19–32, 2005

Nasrallah H, Meyer JM, Goff DC, et al: Low rates of treatment for hypertension, dyslipidemia and diabetes in schizophrenia: data from the CATIE schizophrenia trial sample at baseline. Schizophr Res 86(1–3):15–22, 2006

Nathan DM, Buse JB, Davidson MB, et al: Medical management of hyperglycemia in type 2 diabetes: a consensus algorithm for the initiation and adjustment of therapy. a consensus statement of the American Diabetes Association and the European Association for the Study of Diabetes. Diabetes Care 32(1):193–203, 2009

National Heart, Lung and Blood Institute: Clinical Guidelines on the Identification, Evaluation, and Treatment of Overweight and Obesity in Adults. Bethesda, MD, National Heart, Lung and Blood Institute, 1998

Rose J, Behm F: Adapting smoking cessation treatment according to initial response to precessation nicotine patch. Am J Psychiatry 170(8):860–867, 2013

Sidhu D, Naugler C: Fasting time and lipid levels in a community-based population: a cross-sectional study. Arch Intern Med 172(22):1707–1710, 2012

Stead LF, Perera R, Bullen C, et al: Nicotine replacement therapy for smoking cessation. Cochrane Database of Systematic Reviews 2012, Issue 11. Art. No.: CD000146. DOI: 10.1002/14651858.CD000146.pub4.

Stone NJ, Robinson J, Lichtenstein AH, et al: 2013 ACC/AHA guideline on the treatment of blood cholesterol to reduce atherosclerotic cardiovascular risk in adults: a report of the American College of Cardiology/American Heart Association Task Force on Practice Guidelines. J Am Coll Cardiol pii:S0735–S1097, 2013

Stratton I, Adler A, Neil H: Association of glycaemia with macrovascular and microvascular complications of type 2 diabetes (UKPDS 35): prospective observational study. BMJ 321(7258):405-412, 2000

Tsoi DT, Porwal M, Webster A: Interventions for smoking cessation and reduction in individuals with schizophrenia. Cochrane Database of Systematic Reviews 2013, Issue 2. Art. No.: CD007253. DOI: 10.1002/14651858.CD007253.pub3.

UK Prospective Diabetes Study (UKPDS) Group: Effect of intensive blood-glucose control with metformin on complications in overweight patients with type 2 diabetes (UKPDS 34). Lancet 352(9131):837–853, 1998

U.S. Preventive Services Task Force: Screening for high blood pressure: recommendations and rationale. Am J Prev Med 25(2):159–164, 2003

U.S. Preventive Services Task Force: Screening for Lipid Disorders in Adults. Rockville, MD, U.S. Preventive Services Task Force, 2008. Available at: http://www.uspreventiveservicestaskforce.org/uspstf/uspschol.htm. Accessed August 1, 2013.

Van Horn L, McCoin M, Kris-Etherton PM, et al: The evidence for dietary prevention and treatment of cardiovascular disease. J Am Diet Assoc 108(2):287–331, 2008

Vest A, Heneghan H, Schauer P, et al: Surgical management of obesity and the relationship to cardiovascular disease. Circulation 127(8):945–959, 2013

Viera AJ, Neutze DM: Diagnosis of secondary hypertension: an age-based approach. Am Fam Physician 82(12):1471–1478, 2010

Vodnala D, Rubenfire M, Brook RD: Secondary causes of dyslipidemia. Am J Cardiol 110(6):823–825, 2012

Williams J, Anthenelli R: Double-blind, placebo-controlled study evaluating the safety and efficacy of varenicline for smoking cessation in patients with schizophrenia or schizoaffective disorder. J Clin Psychiatry 73(5):654–660, 2012

Williams J, Foulds J: Successful tobacco dependence treatment in schizophrenia. Am J Psychiatry 164(2):222–227, quiz 373, 2007

Wu R-R, Zhao J-P, Jin H, et al: Lifestyle intervention and metformin for treatment of antipsychotic-induced weight gain: a randomized controlled trial. JAMA 299(2):185–193, 2008

Zapawa L, Hughes J, Benowitz N: Cautions and warnings on the US OTC label for nicotine replacement: what's a doctor to do? Addict Disord 36(4):327–332, 2011

Index

Page numbers printed in **boldface** type refer to tables or figures.

special issues of behavioral care in, 24

SCARED. *See* Screen for Child Anxiety Related Emotional Disorders

Schizophrenia

cardiovascular disease and, 142, **143**

case example of, 217–218

diet and medical comorbidity in, 146

dyslipidemias and, 232

exercise and, 147–148

high-risk sexual activity and, 149–150

increased mortality risk in, **143**

metabolic syndrome and, 219

quality of health care and, 153–154

social networks and, 151

substance abuse and, 145

tobacco use and, 144, 156, 181, 247

Schools, and mental health needs of children, 80

Schroeder v. Albaghdadi (2008), 95

Scotland, and diet of schizophrenia patients, 146–147

Screen for Child Anxiety Related Emotional Disorders (SCARED), 70, 78

Screening

community mental health initiatives for children and, 72–73

as core task of collaborative care team, 19–21

for diabetes, 224–225

for hypertension, 239–240

for obesity, 219–220

pediatric primary care and, 70, 78

for tobacco use, 246

Screening, brief intervention, and referral to treatment (SBIRT) model of care, 246

Security, and legal issues, 108

Selective serotonin reuptake inhibitors (SSRIs), side effects of, 152

Self-management

stepped care and, 23

treatment of diabetes and, 226

"Self-medication" hypothesis, for tobacco use, 144–145, 156

Self-soothing, and distress tolerance skills, 34

Serious mental illness (SMI). *See also* Attention-deficit/hyperactivity disorder; Bipolar disorders; Depression; Generalized anxiety disorder; Panic disorder; Personality disorders; Posttraumatic stress disorder; Psychosis and psychotic disorders; Schizophrenia

diabetes and, 223

integrated care and improvement in health status of, 91

need for medical care in public mental health settings, 141–142

obesity and, 218

primary care provider–psychiatrist partnership and improvement in care for, 59

psychiatrists and provision of general medical care for patients with, 106

Sertraline, **49**

SES. *See* Socioeconomic status

Sexual behavior, and adverse health behaviors of patients with serious mental illness, 149–150, 157–158

Shadowing tool, and behavioral health provider, 28

Shared leadership, of collaborative care teams, 56

Side effects, of psychotropic medications, 151–153, 159–162

Simvastatin, **237**

Skin infections, and substance use disorders, **146**

SMI. *See* Serious mental illness

SOAP note (subjective, objective, assessment, plan), and formal consultation, 46